THE CLEVELAND CLINIC FOUNDATION

CREATIVE COOKING for
RENAL DIABETIC DIETS

First Edition June 1987

Published under exclusive license by
Senay Publishing, Inc.
P.O. Box 397
Chesterland, Ohio 44026

Library of Congress Cataloging-in-Publication Data

The Cleveland Clinic Foundation creative cooking for
    renal diabetic diets.

    Includes index.
    1. Diabetic nephropathies--Diet therapy--Recipes.
2. Large type books. I. Ellis, Pat (Pat Weigel)
II. Cleveland Clinic Foundation. Dept. of Nutrition
Services. III. Title: Creative cooking for renal
diabetic diets. [DNLM: 1. Cookery. 2. Diabetic
Diet--popular works. 3. Diabetic Nephropathies--
diet therapy--popular works. WK 819 C635]
RC918.D53C57 1987   641.5'6314   87-4934
ISBN 0-941511-01-4

THE CLEVELAND CLINIC FOUNDATION

CREATIVE COOKING for
RENAL DIABETIC DIETS

by THE CLEVELAND CLINIC FOUNDATION
DEPARTMENT OF NUTRITION SERVICES

Pat Ellis, M.S., R.D.

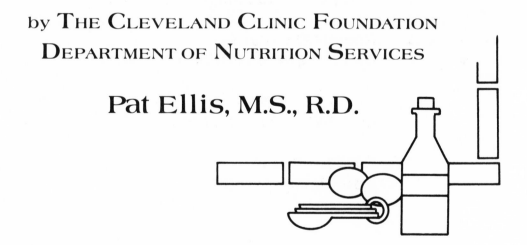

Senay Publishing, Inc.
P.O. Box 397
Chesterland, Ohio 44026

This cookbook has been compiled through the efforts of many individuals at The Cleveland Clinic Foundation. Without the combined contributions and support of these individuals, the publication of this cookbook would not have been possible:

**The Cleveland Clinic Foundation
Dialysis Patients**

**Test Kitchen Staff
Department of Nutrition Services**

**Clinical Dietitians
Department of Nutrition Services**

**Kindy Bontempo
East Side Dialysis Center**

**Ginger Ranallo
Department of Graphic Services**

In Appreciation
The Publisher acknowledges his sincere appreciation to Karen Miller Kovach, M.S., R.D. for her assistance in making this edition possible.

NUTRIENT GUIDELINES FOR RENAL DIABETIC EXCHANGES

FOOD GROUP		CARBO-HYDRATE (G)	PROTEIN (G)	SODIUM (MG)	POTASSIUM (MG)	CALORIES
MEAT		0	8	25	120	75
MILK		6	4	60	175	80
FRUITS		10	1	5	155	40
VEGETABLES		5	1	5	155	20
STARCHES	SALTED	15	2	150	40	75
	UNSALTED	15	2	10	40	75
SALTED FATS		0	0	150	0	100
BEVERAGES		0	0	0	60	0

The exchanges used follow the Renal Diet Instruction Booklet written by the Northern and Eastern Ohio Council on Renal Nutrition.

Special diets are often difficult to follow because they soon become boring and monotonous. **The Cleveland Clinic Foundation Creative Cooking for Renal Diabetic Diets** was written to add variety and imagination to your diet. Favorite everyday and special occasion recipes are given with renal exchanges to make your meals more pleasurable and your diet easier to follow.

Some of these recipes may contain formerly forbidden foods, like nuts, chocolate, sugar or regular cheese. These foods are calculated into the exchanges listed. Use them only as directed. When using food containing sugar, eat them as part of your whole meal, not by themselves. If you need to gain weight, use those recipes which have salted fats. Each salted fat listed adds another 100 calories to the serving. If you are trying to lose weight, either avoid those high calorie dishes or cut back on the margarine and oil. Excess fluid weight gains may mean that you are using too much salt. Substitute salt-free margarine or butter in the recipes, try using salt-free breads and starches (rice, noodles and macaroni) and review your diet instruction to see what salty foods you need to avoid.

The Cleveland Clinic Foundation does not endorse any products or brand names. Recipes specifying brand name ingredients are provided for your convenience. Do not substitute ingredients, unless approved by your dietitian.

CONTENTS

BEVERAGES

FLAVORED COFFEES

VIENNA: 1/3 Cup Instant Coffee
Sugar Substitute to Equal 2/3 Cup Sugar
2/3 Cup "Coffee Mate"
1/2 Teaspoon Cinnamon

ORANGE: 1/2 Cup Instant Coffee
Sugar Substitute to Equal 3/4 Cup Sugar
1 Cup "Coffee Mate"
1/2 Teaspoon Dried Orange Peel

MOCHA: 1/2 Cup Instant Coffee
Sugar Substitute to Equal 1/2 Cup Sugar
1 Cup "Coffee Mate"
2 Tablespoons Unsweetened Cocoa

Blend in blender until powdered. For each serving place 2 rounded teaspoons coffee mix in a cup and add boiling water. Makes 20 servings.

Each serving equals: 1 BEVERAGE

COUNT FLUID AS PART OF DAILY FLUID ALLOWANCE

SPICED TEA

1/2 Cup Loose Tea
1-1/2 Tablespoons Dried Orange or Lemon Peel
1 Tablespoon Whole Cloves
1 Teaspoon Cinnamon

Combine tea, dried peel, cloves and cinnamon. Store in an airtight jar. Place 1 teaspoon tea mix in a tea ball and steep in boiling water to taste.

Each serving equals: 1 BEVERAGE

COUNT FLUID AS PART OF DAILY FLUID ALLOWANCE

HOT COCOA MIX

1 Cup "Coffee Mate"
Sugar Substitute to Equal 3/4 Cup Sugar
6 Tablespoons Unsweetened Cocoa
1/4 Cup Instant Nonfat Dry Milk

Mix all ingredients, store in tightly covered container. To serve, mix 1 tablespoon hot cocoa mix with boiling water to taste. Makes approximately 38 servings.

1 tablespoon mix equals: 1 BEVERAGE

COUNT FLUID AS PART OF DAILY FLUID ALLOWANCE

HOLIDAY EGGNOG

1-1/2 Cups "Coffee Rich"
2 Eggs
2 Tablespoons Sugar
1-1/2 Teaspoons Vanilla

Combine "Coffee Rich", eggs, sugar and vanilla in blender or beat with electric mixer until well mixed. Chill thoroughly. Serve with a generous sprinkle of nutmeg. Makes six 1/3-cup servings.

Each serving equals: **1 UNSALTED STARCH**
                                            80cc FLUID

HOT SPICED WINE

1 Cup Apple Cider
1 Cup Rose' Wine
4 Whole Cloves
1 Stick Cinnamon

Combine ingredients. Simmer to blend flavors. Serve hot. Makes three 2/3-cup servings.

Each serving equals: **1 FRUIT**
                                            160cc FLUID

COOKIES

ALMOND FLAVORED SHORTBREAD

1 Cup Margarine, Softened
1/2 Cup Sugar
2 Teaspoons Almond Extract
2-1/2 Cup Sifted Flour
Sugar

Beat margarine, sugar and almond extract until light and fluffy. Stir in flour and blend well. Refrigerate, covered, for 2 hours. Divide dough in half. Roll out dough, one half at a time, until 1/2-inch thick. Cut with 2-inch cookie cutter. Place cookies on cookie sheet. Make an indentation in the center of each cookie with the handle of a wooden spoon. Bake at 300° for 25 to 30 minutes. Remove from oven and roll in sugar. Cool. Makes 3-1/2 dozen cookies.

Three cookies equal: 1 SALTED STARCH

BROWNIES

1/2 Cup Sifted Flour
1/8 Teaspoon Baking Powder
1/2 Cup Margarine, Softened
1 Cup Sugar

2 Eggs
2 Squares Unsweetened
  Chocolate, Melted
1/2 Teaspoon Vanilla

Mix flour and baking powder; set aside. Cream margarine and sugar until light and fluffy; beat in eggs, 1 at a time, until very light. Beat in melted chocolate and vanilla. Blend in flour mixture just until combined. Pour into lightly greased 8-inch pan, spreading evenly. Bake at 325° for 30 minutes. Cool 10 minutes. With a sharp knife, cut into 12 squares. Cool completely.

Each brownie equals: **1 SALTED STARCH**

BROWNIE MIX

4 Cups Sifted Flour
8 Cups Sugar
2-1/2 Cups Unsweetened Cocoa
4 Teaspoons Baking Powder
2 Cups Shortening

Sift together flour, sugar, cocoa and baking powder into a very large bowl. Cut in shortening with pastry blender or two knives. (You can also do it in several batches with a food processor and then remix it all together.) Store in a covered container in a cool place or refrigerator up to 3 months. Makes about 16 cups.

SHORT-CUT BROWNIES

2 Cups Brownie Mix
2 Eggs, Slightly Beaten
1 Teaspoon Vanilla

Combine mix, eggs and vanilla in a bowl, blending well. Mixture will not be smooth. Spread in a greased 8-inch square baking pan. Bake at 350° for 20 to 25 minutes. Cut into 16 squares.

Each brownie equals: 1 SALTED STARCH

CHRISTMAS SLICES

1 Cup Margarine, at Room Temperature
1/2 Cup Sugar
1 Egg
1/2 Teaspoon Vanilla
2 Cups plus 2 Tablespoons Flour
1/4 Cup (1-1/2 Ounces) Red or Green Tinted Sugar

Beat margarine in a bowl until creamy. Add 1/2 cup sugar, 1/4 cup at a time, beating well after each addition. Add egg and vanilla, beat until light and fluffy. Mix in flour. Cut dough in half. Using lightly floured hands and board; roll each piece into a cylinder about 9 inches long and 1-1/2 inches in diameter. Sprinkle 2 tablespoons of colored sugar on a strip of waxed paper. Using the waxed paper as a sling, gently roll each piece of dough back and forth until it is evenly coated with sugar. (Cylinders now will be approximately 12 inches long, 1 inch in diameter). Wrap dough and chill 6 hours or more. Slice dough as thin as possible then place slices 1 inch apart on ungreased cookie sheets. Bake at 350° for 6 to 8 minutes, until just firm to the touch, but not browned. Remove from oven and transfer to wire racks to cool. Makes about 110 cookies.

Six cookies equal: 1 SALTED STARCH

JAM BARS

1-1/2 Cups Flour
1/2 Cup Sugar
1/2 Teaspoon Baking Powder
1/2 Cup Margarine
1 Egg

1/4 Cup Milk
1/2 Teaspoon Almond Extract
1 Cup Dietetic Strawberry or
Raspberry Jam

Mix flour, sugar and baking powder together, cut margarine into dry ingredients until the mixture has the texture of cornmeal. Add egg, milk and almond extract; mix well. Spread 2/3 of the batter in a 9 x 13-inch pan. Top evenly with jam and drop remaining batter by spoonsful on top. Bake at 400° for 30 minutes. Cool in pan. Cut into 28 bars.

Two bars equal: **1 SALTED STARCH**

LEMON DROPS

1/2 Cup Margarine
1 Cup Sugar
2 Eggs
1 Teaspoon Vanilla
2 Cups Flour
1/2 Teaspoon Baking Soda
1/4 Cup Lemon Juice

Cream margarine and sugar until light and fluffy. Add eggs and vanilla and beat well. Mix flour and baking soda; add with lemon juice to margarine mixture. Mix well. Drop by teaspoonsful onto cookie sheet. Bake at 375° for 10-12 minutes. Makes 3 dozen.

Two cookies equal: 1 SALTED STARCH

MELTAWAYS

1 Cup Margarine
1/2 Cup Sifted Confectioners'
  Sugar
1-1/2 Cups Flour
1 Teaspoon Vanilla
3/4 Cup Finely Chopped Walnuts*
1 Cup Sifted Confectioners' Sugar

In a large bowl, beat margarine with 1/2 cup confectioners' sugar until light and fluffy. Stir in flour, vanilla and nuts, blending well to make a stiff dough. Roll dough, a level teaspoon at a time, into balls between palms of hands. Place 1 inch apart on cookie sheets. Bake at 350° for 15 minutes or until firm. Remove carefully from cookie sheets; while still hot, roll again in 1 cup confectioners' sugar to make a generous white coating. Makes 6 dozen cookies.

Two cookies equal: 1 SALTED STARCH

*Walnuts are high in potassium. They have been specially calculated into this recipe. Use only as directed.

PINEAPPLE COOKIES

6 Tablespoons Margarine
1/2 Cup Sugar
1 Egg
1/2 Cup Undrained Crushed Pineapple (Regular)
1-1/2 Cups Flour
1/4 Teaspoon Baking Soda

Beat margarine with sugar and egg until fluffy. Stir in pineapple. Mix flour and baking soda; add to margarine mixture. Beat well. Drop by teaspoonsful on cookie sheet. Bake at 350° for 10-12 minutes. Makes 3 dozen.

Three cookies equal: **1 SALTED STARCH**

RICH ALMOND COOKIES

1 Cup Margarine, Softened
1/2 Cup Sugar
2 Egg Yolks
2 Tablespoons Water
1-1/2 Teaspoons Almond Extract
2-1/2 Cups Sifted Flour

Cream margarine until fluffy. Gradually add sugar and cream together until light and fluffy. Thoroughly mix in egg yolks, water, almond extract and flour. (Dough may be tinted with food color if desired). Force dough through cookie press onto ungreased cookie sheets. Bake at 500° until golden, about 7-10 minutes. Makes 7 dozen cookies.

Five cookies equal: 1 SALTED STARCH

SCOTTISH SHORTBREAD

1 Cup Margarine, Softened
1/2 Cup Sugar
1/2 Teaspoon Vanilla
2-1/2 Cups Flour

Line the bottoms of two 8-inch round cake pans with waxed paper and set aside. Cream margarine, sugar and vanilla until light and fluffy. Beat in flour, 1/2 cup at a time, until well mixed. Divide dough in half, pat each half evenly into pans. Prick dough all over with a fork to prevent bubbles from forming during baking. Bake for 1 hour at 275° until pale and golden. (Do not brown). Cool in pans for 10 minutes, then remove from pans and cut each into 8 wedges. Makes 16 cookies.

Each cookie equals: 1 SALTED STARCH

SNICKERDOODLES

1 Cup Margarine	2 Teaspoons Cream of Tartar
1-1/2 Cups Sugar	1 Teaspoon Baking Soda
2 Eggs	2 Tablespoons Sugar
2-3/4 Cups Flour	2 Teaspoons Cinnamon

Cream margarine and 1-1/2 cups sugar until light and fluffy. Add eggs and beat well. Mix flour, cream of tartar and baking soda. Add to margarine mixture, mix well. Form into 1-1/4-inch balls. Roll in mixture of 2 tablespoons sugar and 2 teaspoons cinnamon. Place on cookie sheets. Bake at 400° for 8-10 minutes. Makes 5 dozen.

Two cookies equal: **1 SALTED STARCH**

THUMBPRINT COOKIES

1 Teaspoon Vanilla	1 Egg Yolk
1/4 Teaspoon Lemon Extract	1 Cup Sifted Flour
1/2 Cup Margarine	Dietetic Raspberry Jam
1/4 Cup Sugar	

Cream vanilla and lemon extract into margarine. Add sugar gradually; beat in egg yolk. Stir in flour. Shape into small balls. Place on cookie sheet and make a dent in each cookie with floured thumb. Fill "dents" with 1/2 teaspoon jam. Bake at 400° for 15 minutes. Makes 24 cookies.

Three cookies equal: **1 SALTED STARCH**

TEA CAKES

1 Cup Margarine, Softened
1/2 Cup Confectioners' Sugar
1 Tablespoon Water
1 Teaspoon Vanilla
2-1/4 Cups Sifted Flour

Cream margarine and confectioners' sugar until light and fluffy. Add water and vanilla, mix well. Gradually add flour, beating until well mixed. Chill dough for 30 minutes or until firm. Roll dough into 1-inch balls. Place on cookie sheets. Bake at 400° for 10 minutes or until light brown on bottom. Cool. Makes 4 dozen cookies.

Three cookies equal: **1 SALTED STARCH**

QUICK BREADS

HAWAIIAN QUICK BREAD

1/3 Cup Sugar
1/3 Cup Margarine
2 Eggs
2 Cups Flour

3 Teaspoons Baking Powder
1 Cup Crushed Pineapple, Undrained

Beat sugar and margarine until light and fluffy. Add eggs and mix well. Mix flour and baking powder together. Combine sugar and flour mixtures. Blend. Add pineapple, mix to combine. Pour into greased 9 x 5-inch pan. Bake at 350° for 1 hour. Cut into 20 slices.

Each slice equals: **1 SALTED STARCH**

HOLIDAY CRANBERRY BREAD

2 Cups Flour
1 Cup Sugar
1 Tablespoon Orange Peel
1-1/2 Teaspoons Baking Powder
1/2 Teaspoon Baking Soda

3/4 Cup Orange Juice
2 Tablespoons Melted Margarine
1 Egg
1 Cup Chopped Cranberries
1/2 Cup Chopped Nuts*

Combine flour, sugar, orange peel, baking powder and baking soda. Add orange juice, margarine and egg. Mix quickly. Stir in cranberries and nuts. Pour into greased 9 x 5-inch loaf pan. Bake at 325° for 45 to 55 minutes. Slice into 20 slices.

Each slice equals: **1 SALTED STARCH**

* Nuts are high in potassium. They have been specially calculated into this recipe. Use only as directed.

LEMON TEA BREAD

2 Cups Flour
1-1/2 Teaspoons Baking Powder
1/2 Cup Margarine
1 Cup Sugar
2 Eggs
1/3 Cup Milk

1/2 Cup Walnuts*
2 Teaspoons Lemon Peel

Mix flour and baking powder; set aside. Beat margarine and sugar until light and fluffy. Add eggs one at a time, beating well after each addition; beat until light and fluffy. Mix in flour and milk alternately; beat just until combined. Stir in nuts and lemon peel. Spoon into greased 9 x 5-inch loaf pan. Bake at 350° for 55 to 60 minutes or until done. Cut into 20 slices.

Each slice equals: 1 SALTED STARCH

* Walnuts are high in potassium. They have been specially calculated into this recipe. Use only as directed.

PUMPKIN BREAD

2 Cups Flour
2 Teaspoons Baking Powder
1/2 Teaspoon Baking Soda
1 Teaspoon Cinnamon
1/2 Teaspoon Nutmeg

1 Cup Pumpkin
1 Cup Sugar
1/2 Cup Milk
2 Eggs
1/4 Cup Margarine, Softened

Combine flour, baking powder, baking soda, cinnamon and nutmeg. Mix pumpkin, sugar, milk and eggs together in mixing bowl. Add dry ingredients and softened margarine, mix until well blended. Spread in well greased 9 x 5-inch loaf pan. Bake at 350° for 55 minutes or until done. Cut into 20 slices.

Each slice equals: 1 SALTED STARCH

ZUCCHINI BREAD

1-1/2 Cups Flour
1 Teaspoon Cinnamon
1/2 Teaspoon Baking Soda
1/2 Teaspoon Baking Powder
1 Cup Sugar
1/2 Cup Oil

2 Eggs
2 Teaspoons Lemon Peel
1 Cup Grated, Unpeeled Zucchini
1/4 Cup Raisins
1/2 Cup Chopped Walnuts*

Mix flour, cinnamon, baking soda and baking powder together. Combine sugar, oil and eggs in large mixing bowl, mix until smooth. Combine lemon peel, zucchini, raisins and walnuts in separate mixing bowl. Add dry ingredients to sugar mixture. Mix until smooth. Add zucchini mixture and stir until well mixed. Pour into greased and floured 9 x 5-inch pan. Bake at 350° 60 minutes or until done. Cool 10 minutes, remove from pan and continue cooling on wire rack. Cut into 20 slices.

Each slice equals: 1 SALTED STARCH

*Walnuts are high in potassium. They have been specially calculated into this recipe. Use them only as directed.

HOT MUFFINS

1-1/2 Cups Flour   1 Egg
2 Teaspoons Baking Powder   1 Cup Milk
1/2 Cup Sugar   1/4 Cup Oil

Mix flour, baking powder and sugar. Beat egg until frothy, stir in milk and oil. Pour milk mixture into flour mixture, stir quickly just until mixed (batter will still be lumpy). Fill 16 muffin cups equally. Bake at 425° for 25 minutes or until done. Serve hot. Makes 16 muffins.

Each muffin equals: 1 UNSALTED STARCH

APPLE MUFFINS

Make hot muffins, add 1/2 teaspoon cinnamon with flour and 1 cup grated raw (unpared) apple with shortening. Sprinkle muffins with mixture of 2 tablespoons sugar and 1/2 teaspoon cinnamon and bake. Makes 16 muffins.

Each muffin equals: 1 UNSALTED STARCH

JELLY-FILLED MUFFINS

Make hot muffins, fill muffin cups half full. Top with a teaspoon of dietetic jelly. Top with remaining batter and bake. Makes 16 muffins.

Each muffin equals: 1 UNSALTED STARCH

BLUEBERRY CAKE MUFFINS

2 Cups Flour
1-1/2 Teaspoons Baking Powder
1/2 Cup Margarine, Softened
3/4 Cup Sugar

2 Eggs
1 Teaspoon Vanilla
1/2 Cup Milk
1 Cup Blueberries

Preheat oven to 375°. Line 18 muffin cups with paper liners. Mix flour with baking powder and set aside. In a large bowl beat margarine, sugar, eggs and vanilla until light and fluffy. Add milk and flour mixture. Beat just until smooth. Gently fold in blueberries (drain well if canned). Divide muffin batter evenly into muffin cups. Bake 20 to 25 minutes, until golden brown. Makes 18 muffins.

Each muffin equals: 1 SALTED STARCH

CORN MUFFINS

1 Cup Flour
2 Tablespoons Sugar
3 Teaspoons Baking Powder
1 Cup Yellow Cornmeal

1 Egg, Beaten
1/4 Cup Oil
1 Cup Milk

Line 18 muffin cups with paper liners. Mix flour, sugar, baking powder and cornmeal in large bowl. In medium bowl, mix egg, oil and milk. Pour milk mixture into flour mixture all at once; stir quickly with fork until all ingredients are just moistened (batter will be lumpy). Quickly dip batter into muffin pans. Bake at 425° for 15 minutes or until golden. Serve hot.

Each muffin equals: **1 SALTED STARCH**

STREUSEL-TOPPED MUFFINS

TOPPING:
- 1/4 Cup Brown Sugar*
- 1/4 Cup Flour
- 2 Tablespoons Margarine
- 2 Teaspoons Cinnamon

BATTER:
- 1-1/3 Cup Flour
- 1-1/2 Teaspoons Baking Powder
- 1/4 Cup Margarine
- 1/2 Cup Sugar
- 1 Egg
- 1/2 Cup Milk

Preheat oven to 375°. Line 14 muffin cups with paper liners.

Make Topping: Mix brown sugar, flour, margarine, and cinnamon until crumbly.

Make Batter: Mix flour and baking powder, set aside. Beat margarine until fluffy, beat in sugar. Add the egg and beat until light and fluffy. Blend in milk, then flour, just until combined. Divide evenly into 14 muffin cups. Sprinkle topping over each muffin. Bake 15 to 18 minutes. Cool slightly, serve warm. Makes 14 muffins.

Each muffin equals: 1 SALTED STARCH

* Brown sugar has been specially calculated into this recipe.
  Use only as directed.

BAKING POWDER BISCUITS

2 Cups Flour
3 Teaspoons Baking Powder
1/3 Cup Shortening
3/4 Cup Milk

Mix flour and baking powder, cut in shortening until mixture resembles coarse oatmeal. Pour in milk and stir quickly with a fork. Turn dough out on lightly floured board, knead 10 times. Gently roll out dough and cut into 12 biscuits. Bake at 450° for 10 to 12 minutes or until golden brown.

Each biscuit equals: 1 SALTED STARCH

BISCUIT MIX

3 Cups Flour
2 Tablespoons Baking Powder
1/3 Cup Shortening

Mix ingredients until thoroughly combined. Store tightly in refrigerator. Makes 3-3/4 cups. Keeps at least 4 weeks in the refrigerator.

QUICK BISCUITS

1/4 to 1/3 Cup Milk
1 Cup Biscuit Mix

Add milk to biscuit mix and stir with a fork. Dough should be soft and slightly sticky. Knead on floured surface about 10 times. Roll out and cut into 6 biscuits. Bake 10 to 12 minutes at 450° until golden brown.

Each biscuit equals: 1 SALTED STARCH

APPLE CHEESE-FILLED ROLLS

2 Cups Biscuit Mix (See Recipe Page C 10)
1 Cup Sour Cream
One 8-Ounce Package Cream Cheese, Softened
1/3 Cup Sugar
1 Tablespoon Grated Orange Rind
1-1/2 Cups Thinly Sliced, Pared Apples
1/4 Cup Confectioners' Sugar
1-2 Teaspoons Orange Juice

Mix biscuit mix and sour cream until soft dough forms. Turn dough out onto floured board and kneed until smooth, about 20 times. Divide in half. Roll each half into a 9-inch square. Cut into nine 3-inch squares. Place on cookie sheets. Mix cream cheese, sugar and orange peel. Place 2 apple slices on center of each square; top with 1 tablespoon cream cheese mixture. Bring 2 opposite corners of dough to center of each square, overlapping tightly, pinch well. Bake at 400°, until crust is golden brown, approximately 12 to 15 minutes. Cool slightly and drizzle with mixture of confectioners' sugar and orange juice. Makes 18 rolls.

Each roll equals: **1 SALTED STARCH**

ONION PARSLEY BUTTERFINGERS

2 Cups Biscuit Mix (See Recipe Page C 10)
1 Egg
1/2 Cup Milk
1/2 Cup Margarine
2 Tablespoons Onion Flakes
1 Tablespoon Parsley

Combine biscuit mix, egg and milk; beat vigorously 20 strokes. Turn dough out on lightly floured surface and knead lightly 1/2 minute; roll out in 12 x 8-inch rectangle and cut with floured knife in 3 x 1-inch fingers. Melt margarine in jelly-roll pan in 450° oven. Lay fingers in margarine; turn once to coat both sides and arrange side by side in pan. Sprinkle with mixture of onion and parsley flakes and bake about 8 minutes or until golden brown. Remove to rack. Serve warm. Makes 32.

Two butterfingers equal: 1 SALTED STARCH

BLUEBERRY KUCHEN

2 Tablespoons Margarine
1/2 Cup Sugar
1 Egg
1/2 Cup Milk
1 Cup Flour
2 Teaspoons Baking Powder

1 Teaspoon Vanilla
1 Cup Blueberries
1/2 Cup Flour
1/4 Cup Sugar
1/4 Cup Margarine

Cream 2 tablespoons margarine and 1/2 cup sugar; add egg, beat well. Add milk, 1 cup flour, baking powder and vanilla and mix well. Pour batter into greased 8 x 8-inch pan. Sprinkle blueberries (drain well, if canned) over batter. Combine 1/2 cup flour, 1/4 cup sugar and 1/4 cup margarine until crumbly. Sprinkle over blueberries. Bake at 375° for 25 to 30 minutes. Cut into 16 pieces.

Each piece equals: **1 SALTED STARCH**

GERMAN COFFEE CAKE

BATTER:
- 1 Cup Flour
- 1/3 Cup Sugar
- 1/8 Teaspoon Nutmeg
- 2 Teaspoons Baking Powder
- 1/2 Cup Milk
- 1 Egg
- 2 Tablespoons Margarine, Melted

TOPPING:
- 3 Tablespoons Flour
- 1/2 Teaspoon Cinnamon
- 1/3 Cup Brown Sugar*
- 3 Tablespoons Margarine, Melted

Mix 1 cup flour, sugar, nutmeg and baking powder. Add milk, egg and 2 tablespoons margarine. Mix well. Pour into 9 x 9-inch greased baking dish. Mix 3 tablespoons flour, cinnamon, brown sugar and 3 tablespoons margarine. Spoon over batter, making indentations into batter so some of the topping sinks down into coffee cake. Bake at 350° for 20 to 25 minutes. Serve warm. Makes 12 servings.

Each serving equals: 1 SALTED STARCH

* Brown sugar is high in potassium. It has been specially calculated into this recipe. Use only as directed.

POPOVER PANCAKE

1/4 Cup Margarine
1/2 Cup Flour
1/2 Cup Milk
2 Eggs
Dash Cinnamon or Nutmeg

Melt margarine in pie pan. Beat flour, milk, eggs and cinnamon or nutmeg until smooth. Pour into pie pan containing margarine. Bake at 375° for 15 minutes until lightly browned. Serve with artificially sweetened fruit or dietetic pancake syrup. (Strawberries are best.) Makes 2 servings.

Each serving equals: **1 OUNCE MEAT**
                            2 UNSALTED STARCHES

HUNGARIAN PANCAKES

1 Egg
3/4 Cup Flour
2 Cups "Coffee Rich"
1 Teaspoon Sugar
1 Teaspoon Margarine

Mix egg, flour, "Coffee Rich" and sugar together well with rotary beater. Let batter stand 30 minutes. Melt 1 teaspoon margarine in 9-inch skillet, coat the bottom of the pan lightly. Pour 1/4 cup batter into hot skillet. Quickly tip skillet so batter covers the bottom of the whole pan. Cook over low heat until browned on one side. Transfer to warm plate. Spread with dietetic jam, or dietetic pancake syrup. Roll up. Repeat with remaining batter, adding more margarine as needed. Serve at once. Makes 10 pancakes.

One pancake equals: **1 UNSALTED STARCH**

PANCAKES

1 Cup Flour
2 Teaspoons Baking Powder
2 Tablespoons Sugar

1 Egg, Beaten
1 Cup Milk
3 Tablespoons Margarine, Melted

Mix flour, baking powder and sugar. Mix beaten egg, milk and melted margarine. Pour into flour mixture all at once. Mix until just combined (batter will be lumpy). Heat skillet or griddle to 425°. Use a scant 1/4 cup batter for each pancake. Makes ten 4-inch pancakes. Serve with margarine and dietetic pancake syrup.

One pancake equals: 1 SALTED STARCH

BLUEBERRY PANCAKES

Add 1 cup blueberries (drain, if canned) to pancake batter, fold in carefully, being careful not to break the berries. Cook and serve as directed above.

FRENCH TOAST

2 Eggs
3/4 Cup Milk
6 Slices Bread

Mix egg and milk together and pour into a shallow bowl. Dip slices of bread into mixture, turn to coat. Grill both sides for a few minutes on a hot greased grill or skillet until golden brown. Serve with margarine and dietetic pancake syrup. Makes 6 slices.

Each slice equals: **1/2 OUNCE MEAT**
1 SALTED STARCH

Extra french toast can be placed on a cookie sheet, cooled and frozen for a few hours. After french toast is frozen, place it in a plastic bag. Thaw and heat individual slices in your toaster.

SPICED FRENCH TOAST

Add 1 teaspoon vanilla, 1/4 teaspoon nutmeg, and 1/4 teaspoon cinnamon to milk and egg mixture in french toast recipe above and proceed as directed.

DESSERTS

2-CRUST PIE SHELL

2 Cups Sifted Flour
3/4 Cup Shortening
4 to 5 Tablespoons Ice Water

Cut shortening into flour until mixture resembles coarse cornmeal. Quickly sprinkle ice water, 1 tablespoon at a time, tossing lightly with a fork. (Pastry should be moist enough to hold together, not sticky). Shape pastry into a ball, cover and refrigerate until ready to use.

Divide pastry in half. Roll out to 11-inch circle and place in pan. Turn prepared filling into pan. Roll out top crust, make several gashes near center for steam vents, place on filling, crimp edges and bake as directed.

1-CRUST PIE SHELL

1 Cup Flour
1/3 Cup, Plus 1 Tablespoon Shortening
2 to 2-1/2 Tablespoons Ice Water

Follow directions for 2-crust pie shell above. Roll out to 11-inch circle and place in pan.

If pie and filling are not to be baked together, prick bottom and sides well with fork. Bake at 450° for 10 to 12 minutes or until golden.

GRAHAM CRACKER PIE SHELL

8 Large Graham Cracker Rectangles, Crushed
2 Tablespoons Sugar
1/4 Cup Margarine, Melted

Combine crushed graham crackers, sugar and melted margarine. Pat into a 9-inch pie pan, evenly covering bottom and sides of pan. Chill for 1 hour or bake at 350° for 10 minutes and cool before filling.

STRAWBERRY
CREAM CHEESE PIE

Graham Cracker Crust
  (See recipe above)
2 Cups Fresh Strawberries, Hulled
3 Tablespoons Sugar
One 8-Ounce Package Cream Cheese, Softened
1/2 Teaspoon Vanilla
2 Cups "Cool Whip"

Prepare graham cracker crust according to recipe, using 9-inch pie pan. Arrange whole strawberries (pointing up) in bottom of crust. Save several berries for garnish. Gradually add sugar to cream cheese in bowl, blending well. Add vanilla. Fold in "Cool Whip" and spoon into pie shell over berries. Chill at least 3 hours. Garnish with remaining berries. Makes 10 servings.

Each serving equals: **1 SALTED STARCH**
                             1/2 FRUIT

LIGHT AND FRUITY PIE

Graham Cracker Crust
  (See Recipe Page D 2)
One 3-Ounce Package Artificially Sweetened Gelatin Dessert
2/3 Cup Boiling Water
2 Cups Ice Cubes
One 8-Ounce Container "Cool Whip"
1 Cup Fruit (Use 1 Cup Diced Fresh Strawberries, Blueberries or
  Raspberries or Canned, Drained, Crushed Pineapple)

Prepare graham cracker crust in 9-inch pie pan as directed. Dissolve gelatin in boiling water, stirring constantly about 3 minutes. Add ice cubes and stir until gelatin is thickened, about 2 to 3 minutes. Remove any unmelted ice. Blend in "Cool Whip" stir until smooth. Fold in fruit. Chill until mixture mounds. Spoon into pie crust. Chill 3 hours. Cut into 8 pieces.

Each serving equals: **1 SALTED STARCH**
                                    1/2 FRUIT

SWEET CHOCOLATE CREAM PIE

Graham Cracker Crust (See Recipe Page D 2)
4 Ounces Sweet Chocolate
1/3 Cup Milk
1 Tablespoons Sugar
One 3-Ounce Package Cream Cheese, Softened
2 Cups "Cool Whip"

Prepare graham cracker crust; set aside. Make several chocolate curls from chocolate with sharp knife; set aside for garnish. Heat chocolate and 2 tablespoons milk over low heat, stirring until melted. Beat sugar into cream cheese; add remaining milk and chocolate mixture. Beat until smooth. Fold "Cool Whip" into chocolate mixture. Blend until smooth. Spoon mixture into crust. Freeze about 4 hours. Garnish with chocolate curls. Makes 10 servings.

Each serving equals: 1 UNSALTED STARCH
                        1/2 FRUIT

IMPOSSIBLE PUMPKIN PIE

2 Eggs
1/2 Cup Sugar
2 Cups "Coffee Rich"
1/4 Teaspoon Cloves
1/2 Teaspoon Ginger
1/4 Teaspoon Nutmeg
1 Teaspoon Cinnamon
1-1/2 Cups Pumpkin
1/2 Cup Biscuit Mix
   (See Recipe Page C 10)

Blend all ingredients in blender. Pour into greased 9-inch pie pan. Bake at 350° for 50 to 60 minutes. Let stand 15 minutes. Makes 8 servings.

Each serving equals: 1 SALTED STARCH
                        1 FRUIT

EASY LAYER CAKE

2 Cups Sifted Cake Flour*   1 Cup Milk
1 Cup Sugar   1 Egg
2-1/2 Teaspoons Baking Powder   1 Teaspoon Vanilla
1/3 Cup Margarine

Mix flour, sugar and baking powder. Add margarine and milk; beat at medium speed with electric mixer for 2 minutes. Add egg and vanilla, beat 2 minutes more. Pour into 2 greased and floured 9-inch cake pans. Bake at 350° for 25 to 30 minutes. Cool in pans 10 minutes. Remove cake from pans and cool thoroughly on wire rack. Cut into 16 pieces.

Each piece equals: 1 SALTED STARCH

* 1-3/4 cup sifted all-purpose flour may be
  substituted for sifted cake flour.

JELLY-ROLL CAKE

4 Eggs
3/4 Cup Sifted Cake Flour
1 Teaspoon Baking Powder
3/4 Cup Sugar
Confectioners' Sugar
1 Cup Dietetic Raspberry Jam

In small bowl, let eggs warm to room temperature, about 1 hour. Lightly grease bottom of 15 x 10 x 1-inch jelly-roll pan; then line bottom with waxed paper. Mix flour and baking powder, set aside. At high speed, beat eggs until very thick and lemon colored. Beat in granulated sugar, 2 tablespoons at a time; continue beating 5 more minutes, or until very thick. Gently fold in flour mixture, just until combined. Turn into prepared pan, spreading evenly. Bake at 400° for 9 minutes or just until surface springs back when gently pressed with fingertip.

Meanwhile, on a clean tea towel, sift confectioners' sugar, forming a 15 x 10-inch rectangle. Invert cake on sugar; gently peel off waxed paper. Starting with narrow end, roll up cake (towel and all). Place, seam side down, on wire rack to cool, about 20 minutes. Gently unroll cake, remove towel. Spread with preserves; roll up again. Place seam side down on serving plate; let stand covered at least 1 hour before serving. To serve, sift confectioners' sugar over top; slice on diagonal. Makes 16 servings.

Each serving equals: 1 UNSALTED STARCH

* 2/3 cup sifted all-purpose flour may be substituted
  for sifted cake flour.

MARBLE LOAF CAKE

1-1/2 Squares Unsweetened Chocolate
2-1/2 Cups Sifted Cake Flour*
3 Teaspoons Baking Powder
1/2 Cup Margarine
1-1/2 Cups Sugar
3 Eggs
3/4 Teaspoon Vanilla
3/4 Cup Milk

Melt chocolate over hot, not boiling water. Let cool. Preheat oven to 350°. Grease and flour a 9 x 5-inch loaf pan (or two 8-inch layer pans). Mix flour and baking powder. Set aside. Beat margarine and sugar until light, add eggs and vanilla, beating until very light and fluffy. Beat in flour mixture (in fourths), alternately with milk (in thirds), beginning and ending with flour mixture. In a medium bowl, combine about one-third batter with chocolate, mixing well. Spoon plain and chocolate batters, alternately, into prepared pan. With knife cut through batter, forming a "Z" to marbleize. Bake 65 minutes for loaf pan, 30-35 minutes for layer pans, until done. Cool in pan 15 minutes, remove and cool thoroughly on wire racks. Cut into 24 slices.

Each slice equals: 1 SALTED STARCH

*2 cups plus 3 tablespoons sifted all-purpose flour may be substituted for sifted cake flour.

TEXAS CAKE

1 Cup Water
1 Cup Margarine
1/4 Cup Unsweetened Cocoa
2 Cups Flour
1-1/2 Cups Sugar
1 Teaspoon Baking Soda
2 Eggs
1/2 Cup Sour Cream

Heat water, margarine and cocoa until margarine is melted. Mix flour, sugar, baking soda, eggs and sour cream into cocoa mixture. Pour into ungreased 15 x 10 x 1-inch jelly-roll pan (batter is thin.) Bake at 350° for 20 minutes. Cut into 30 slices.

Each serving equals: **1 SALTED STARCH**

WESTERN GINGERBREAD

1 Cup Milk
1 Tablespoon Lemon Juice
2 Cups Flour
1-1/4 Cup Sugar
1 Teaspoon Baking Powder
1 Teaspoon Cinnamon

1-1/2 Teaspoon Ginger
1/2 Cup Margarine
1 Egg
2 Tablespoons Molasses*
1 Teaspoon Baking Soda
1 Tablespoon Margarine

Mix milk and lemon juice. Let stand. Mix flour, sugar, baking powder, cinnamon and ginger. Cut in 1/2 cup margarine until fine. Reserve 1/2 cup of crumb mixture for topping. Add baking soda to milk mixture and dissolve. To remaining crumbs, add egg, molasses and milk mixture. Beat with electric mixer for 2 minutes on low speed. Pour into greased 13 x 9-inch pan. Cut 1 tablespoon margarine into reserved crumb mixture. Sprinkle over batter. Bake at 350° for 30-35 minutes. Cut into 24 pieces.

Each piece equals: **1 SALTED STARCH**

* Molasses is high in potassium. It has been specially calculated in this recipe. Use only as directed.

BANANA SPLIT DESSERT

6 Whole Graham Crackers, Crushed
2 Tablespoon Margarine, Melted
1 Egg
1/4 Cup Margarine
1/2 Cup Confectioners' Sugar
1 Cup Undrained, Crushed Pineapple (Regular)
1 Medium Banana, Thinly Sliced
2 Cups "Cool Whip"

Combine graham cracker crumbs and margarine. Pat into an 8-inch square pan. Set aside. Combine egg, margarine and confectioners' sugar; beat for 15 minutes. Pour over crust. Top with crushed pineapple and banana slices. Spread "Cool Whip" on top. Makes 9 servings.

Each serving equals: 1 SALTED STARCH
**   1/2 FRUIT**

FROZEN CHOCOLATE CHIP CHEESECAKE

1-1/4 Cups Crushed Graham Crackers (16 Squares)
2 Tablespoons Sugar
6 Tablespoons Margarine, Melted
One 8-Ounce Package
  Plus One 3-Ounce Package Cream Cheese, Softened
1 Quart Chocolate Ice Cream
1/2 Cup Semisweet Chocolate Chips, Chopped

Combine graham cracker crumbs, sugar and margarine. Press on the bottom and 1-3/4-inches up the sides of an 8-inch spring-form pan. Chill. Beat cream cheese with electric mixer, until fluffy. Set aside. Stir ice cream just enough to soften, gradually add to cream cheese, beating with mixer until smooth. Fold in chopped chocolate chips (save a tablespoon for garnish). Pour into crust. Cover and freeze 8 hours or overnight. To serve, let stand at room temperature 30 to 40 minutes. Garnish with reserved chocolate. Makes 10 servings.

Each serving equals: **1 MILK**
                                   1 SALTED STARCH

TROPICAL CHEESECAKE

1/2 Cup Graham Cracker Crumbs
2 Tablespoons Margarine, Melted
One 8-Ounce Package Cream Cheese, Softened
1/2 Cup Sifted Confectioners' Sugar
2-1/2 Cups Crushed Pineapple, Well Drained (Regular)
2 Cups "Cool Whip"

Mix graham cracker crumbs and margarine, reserve 2 tablespoons for garnish. Press crumbs on the bottom of an 8-inch round cake pan; chill. Whip cream cheese and confectioners' sugar until fluffy. Stir in pineapple and "Cool Whip". Spread over crust. Sprinkle with reserved crumbs; chill well. Makes 8 servings.

Each serving equals: **1 SALTED STARCH**
                              1 FRUIT

GLORIFIED RICE

3-1/2 Cups "Cool Whip"
1/2 Teaspoon Vanilla
2 Cups Cooked Rice
2/3 Cup Drained Crushed Pineapple (Regular)

Blend vanilla into "Cool Whip". Combine rice and pineapple; fold into "Cool Whip" and chill. Makes eight generous 1/2-cup servings.

Each serving equals: 1 UNSALTED STARCH

QUICK 'N EASY CHOCOLATE ICE CREAM

2 Cups "Cool Whip", Thawed
1/4 Cup "Hershey's" Chocolate Flavored Syrup, Chilled

Fold chilled chocolate syrup gently into thawed "Cool Whip". Refreeze in container or individual covered serving dishes. Makes 6 servings.

Each serving equals: 1 FRUIT

LIME SNOW

2 Envelopes Unflavored Gelatin
1 Cup Cold Water
1/4 Cup Sugar
One 6-Ounce Can Frozen Limeade Concentrate (Keep Frozen)
1/2 Cup Ice Water
2 Egg Whites

Sprinkle gelatin over cold water in saucepan. Place over low heat; stir constantly until gelatin dissolves, 2 to 3 minutes. Stir in sugar, stir to dissolve. Remove from heat. Add limeade concentrate and ice water; stir until melted. Chill until slightly thicker than consistency of unbeaten egg white. Add egg whites to gelatin mixture, beat until mixture begins to hold its shape. Turn into 6-cup mold. Chill until firm. Unmold. Makes eight 1/2-cup servings.

Each serving equals: 1 UNSALTED STARCH

CRANBERRY NUT PUDDING

2-1/2 Cups Cranberries
  (Fresh or Frozen)
2/3 Cup Brown Sugar*
1/3 Cup Water
6 Tablespoons Margarine, Softened
1/3 Cup Sugar
1 Egg
1/2 Cup Flour
1/4 Teaspoon Allspice
1/3 Cup Chopped Walnuts*

Combine cranberries, brown sugar and water in a saucepan. Bring to a boil and cook, stirring until cranberries pop, about 5 minutes. Divide between eight 6-ounce custard cups, about 1/4 cup each. Beat margarine and sugar until fluffy. Beat in egg. Stir in flour and allspice, fold in walnuts. Spoon batter, about 2 tablespoons each, into berry-filled custard cups, dividing batter evenly. Place custard cups on a cookie sheet. Bake at 350° for 18 to 20 minutes. Serve warm. Makes 8 servings.

Each serving equals: **1 SALTED STARCH**
                            1 FRUIT

* Brown sugar and walnuts have been specially
  calculated into this recipe. Use them only as directed.

MAIN DISHES

MAIN DISHES

MAIN DISHES

MAIN DISHES

BEEF RAGOUT

2 Tablespoons Margarine
1 Pound Lean Beef, Cut in 3/4-Inch Cubes
1/2 Cup Finely Sliced Onions
1/8 Teaspoon Garlic Powder
1 Cup Fresh Mushrooms
   (Slice Stems and Caps Separately)
1 Crumbled Bay Leaf
1 Teaspoon Parsley
1 Teaspoon Rosemary or Oregano
2 Teaspoons Orange Marmalade
Dash of Cinnamon
1/4 Teaspoon Pepper
1/4 Green Pepper, Sliced
1/4 Cup Water

Melt margarine in large skillet. Add beef cubes; brown well on all sides over high heat. Lower heat, add onions, garlic and sliced stems of the mushrooms. Saute until onions are tender. Add bay leaf, parsley, rosemary, marmalade, cinnamon and pepper. Cover and simmer over low heat 1-1/2 hours, or until tender. Check occasionally and add a little water if meat appears dry. Ten minutes before ragout is done, add green pepper and sliced mushroom caps. Cover and complete cooking. Serve over buttered noodles. Makes 5 servings, approximately 1/3 cup each.

Each serving equals: **2 OUNCES MEAT**
                             1 VEGETABLE

BEEF STEAK WITH ONIONS

1 Pound Round Steak, 3/4 Inch Thick
1/4 Cup Flour
1/8 Teaspoon Onion Powder
Dash Garlic Powder
1/4 Teaspoon Pepper
3 Tablespoons Margarine
1/2 Cup Water
3 Cups Finely Sliced Onions
1/4 Teaspoon Paprika

Cut steak into 6 pieces, coat each piece with flour mixed with onion powder, garlic powder and pepper. Brown in hot margarine. Add water, cover and bake at 350° for 1 hour. Top meat with onion slices, sprinkle with paprika. Add a little more water if necessary. Cover and continue cooking until meat is tender, about 30 minutes. Makes 6 servings.

Each serving equals: 2 OUNCES MEAT
                        1 VEGETABLE
                        1 SALTED FAT

BEEF STROGANOFF

2 Cups Fresh Sliced Mushrooms
3/4 Cup Sliced Onions
3 Tablespoons Margarine
1-1/2 Pounds Round Steak
1 Cup Water

1 Teaspoon Dry Mustard
1/8 Teaspoon Pepper
2 Tablespoons Flour
1/4 Cup Water
1 Cup Sour Cream

Saute mushrooms and onions in large skillet in margarine until soft; remove from skillet and set aside. Slice the meat into strips the size of a pencil, 3 to 4 inches long, and brown in skillet. Reduce heat to simmer. Return vegetables to skillet and add 1 cup water, dry mustard and pepper. Cover and simmer 45 minutes or until meat is tender, adding more water if necessary. Combine flour with 1/4 cup water, stir until smooth. Stir into meat mixture and cook until sauce thickens, about 2 minutes. Reduce heat to low. Just before serving, stir in sour cream. Serve over hot buttered noodles. Makes six 1/2-cup servings.

Each serving equals: 3 OUNCES MEAT
                         1 VEGETABLE

EGGPLANT AND GROUND BEEF CASSEROLE

3/4 Pound Fresh Eggplant
1/2 Cup Flour
1 Egg
1 Tablespoon Milk
1/4 Cup Dry Bread Crumbs
1/8 Teaspoon Garlic Powder
3 Tablespoons Oil
1/2 Pound Ground Beef

2 Tablespoons Tomato Paste
  (Canned Without Salt)
6 Tablespoons Water
1/2 Cup Mozzarella Cheese,
  Grated*
1 Teaspoon Parsley
1/4 Teaspoon Pepper

Peel eggplant and cut in 1/2-inch slices. Stack between paper towels and press out moisture. Coat with flour, dip in a mixture of beaten egg and milk. Coat again with bread crumbs. Heat oil and garlic powder, add eggplant a few slices at a time and brown on both sides. Add more oil if necessary. Drain eggplant on paper towels. Brown meat in same pan, drain off fat. Add tomato paste, water, cheese, parsley and pepper; stir to combine. Arrange eggplant slices and meat mixture in alternate layers in a small casserole, ending with meat sauce on top. Bake at 375° for 45 minutes. Makes 4 servings.

Each serving equals: 2 OUNCES MEAT
                                1 UNSALTED STARCH
                                1 VEGETABLE
                                1 SALTED FAT

* Mozzarella cheese does contain salt. It has been specially calculated into this recipe. Use it only as directed.

GOURMET HAMBURGERS

1/2 Cup Minced Onions
2 Tablespoons Margarine
1 Pound Ground Beef
1/8 Teaspoon Pepper
Dash Thyme
1 Tablespoon Margarine
1/2 Cup Red Wine
1 Teaspoon Margarine

Saute onions in 2 tablespoons margarine until onions are tender. Mix onions with ground beef, pepper and thyme. Divide into 5 patties and pan fry in 1 tablespoon margarine until done to taste. Remove hamburgers to hot platter and deglaze the pan with red wine. Scrape up all pan juices and brownings and cook until reduced by half. Remove from heat, add 1 teaspoon margarine. Stir briefly and pour over hamburgers. Serves 5.

Each hamburger equals: **2 OUNCES MEAT**
                               1/2 VEGETABLE
                               1 SALTED FAT

ITALIAN PIE

3/4 Pound Ground Beef
1/4 Cup Chopped Onion
1/8 Teaspoon Garlic Powder
1/2 Cup Small Curd Creamed Cottage Cheese*
1/4 Cup Grated Parmesan Cheese*
1 Teaspoon Oregano
1/2 Teaspoon Basil
One 6-Ounce Can Tomato Paste (Canned Without Salt)
3/4 Cup (3 Ounces) Shredded Mozzarella Cheese
1 Cup "Coffee Rich"
2/3 Cup Biscuit Mix (See Recipe Page C 10)
2 Eggs
1/4 Teaspoon Pepper

Saute ground beef with onion and garlic powder until browned, drain. Lightly grease pie pan. Layer cottage cheese and parmesan cheese in pie pan. Mix cooked beef, oregano, basil, tomato paste and 1/2 cup mozzarella cheese; spoon evenly over top. Beat "Coffee Rich", biscuit mix, eggs and pepper until smooth. Pour into pie plate. Bake at 400° for 30 to 35 minutes, until golden brown and knife inserted halfway between center and edge comes out clean. Sprinkle with remaining mozzarella cheese. Let stand 5 minutes before cutting. Cut into 6 servings.

Each serving equals: **2 OUNCES MEAT**
                                  1 SALTED STARCH
                                  1 VEGETABLE

* Cottage, parmesan and mozzarella cheese do contain added salt. They have been specially calculated into this recipe. Use only as directed.

LASAGNA

2 Tablespoons Oil
1/2 Cup Finely Chopped Onion
1/8 Teaspoon Garlic Powder
1 Pound Ground Beef
1 Pound Canned Salt-Free Tomatoes
One 6-Ounce Can Tomato Paste (Canned Without Salt)
1/2 Cup Water
1/2 Teaspoon Pepper
1/4 Teaspoon Basil
1/2 Teaspoon Fennel
1 Teaspoon Parsley
2 Teaspoons Sugar
9 Lasagna Noodles (1/2 Pound)
2 Eggs
1 Pound Cottage Cheese*
2 Teaspoon Parsley
1/4 Pound Mozzarella Cheese, Cut in Thin Slices*
1/4 Cup Grated Parmesan Cheese*

In a large heavy pan, saute onion, garlic and ground beef in oil. Stir frequently, breaking up ground beef, until beef is well browned. Add tomatoes, tomato paste and water, mash tomatoes with a wooden spoon. Add pepper, basil, fennel, 1 teaspoon parsley and sugar. Bring to boil, reduce heat. Cover and simmer, stirring occasionally, until thick, about 1-1/2 hours. In an 8-quart kettle, bring 3 quarts of water to a boil, add lasagna noodles, 2 or 3 at a time. Return to boiling; boil uncovered stirring occasionally, 10 minutes, or just until tender. Drain in colander; rinse under cold water. Dry on paper towels. In a medium bowl, combine eggs, cottage cheese and 2 teaspoons parsley, mix. In

(Continued on next page)

LASAGNA

the bottom of an 8 x 10-inch baking dish, spoon 1/3 sauce, top with 5 noodles, overlapping. Spread with 1/2 of cottage cheese mixture and 1/2 of mozzarella cheese, repeat using remaining 4 noodles, cottage cheese, mozzarella cheese and sauce. Sprinkle with parmesan cheese. Cover with foil, tucking around edge. Bake 25 minutes at 375°, remove foil and bake 20 minutes longer until bubbly. Cool 15 minutes before serving.

Cut into 12 servings, each serving equals:

2 OUNCES MEAT
1 SALTED STARCH
1 VEGETABLE

Cut into 9 servings, each serving equals:

3 OUNCES MEAT
1 SALTED STARCH
1 VEGETABLE

* Cottage cheese, mozzarella and parmesan cheese do contain added salt. They have been specially calculated into this recipe. Use them only as directed.

LONDON BROIL

1 Pound Flank Steak
1-1/2 Teaspoons Oil
1 Teaspoon Lemon Juice

Dash Pepper
Dash Garlic Powder
1 Teaspoon Parsley

Wipe steak dry with paper towels. Combine oil, lemon juice, pepper, garlic powder and parsley; use half to brush on top of steak. Broil, 4 inches from heat, 5 minutes. Turn and brush with rest of the oil mixture and broil 3 to 5 minutes longer. To serve, slice very thin on diagonal across grain. Makes six 2-ounce servings.

Each serving equals: **2 OUNCES MEAT**

MEAT LOAF

2 Eggs, Beaten
1/2 Cup Milk
1/2 Cup Soft Bread Crumbs
1/4 Cup Chopped Onions
2 Tablespoons Chopped
 Green Pepper

1/4 Teaspoon Thyme
1/4 Teaspoon Marjoram
1/4 Teaspoon Pepper
1-1/2 Pounds Ground Beef

Combine all ingredients except ground beef. Add ground beef, mix well. Shape mixture into a loaf, place in a loaf pan. Bake at 350° about 1-1/4 hours. Makes 8 servings.

Each serving equals: **2 OUNCES MEAT**

OVEN DINNER

1 Piece Aluminum Foil, 12 x 15 Inches
1 Medium Potato
1 Small Carrot
1 Medium Slice Onion
3 Ounce Beef Pattie
  (If You Divide 1 Pound of Ground Beef into 5 Patties,
  Each Pattie Will Be Almost 3 Ounces)
Pepper
Parsley
1 Tablespoon Margarine

Early in the day, peel and slice potato and carrot into thin 1/8-inch slices. Soak in a large pan of water. An hour before dinner, place beef pattie in the center of foil, sprinkle with pepper, top with onion slice and drained slices of potato and carrot, sprinkle with more pepper and parsley flakes. Top with margarine. Close tightly. Bake on a cookie sheet for 1 hour at 375°. Serves 1.

Oven dinner equals: **2 OUNCES MEAT**
                             1 VEGETABLES
                             1 UNSALTED STARCH (POTATO)

Limit to 1 Serving Potato a Day.

PIQUANT LIVER AND ONIONS

1 Cup Thinly Sliced Onions
2 Tablespoons Margarine
1/4 Cup Flour
1/8 Teaspoon Pepper
1 Pound Thinly Sliced Liver
2 Tablespoons Margarine
3 Tablespoons Vinegar
1 Teaspoon Parsley

Cook onions in margarine until tender; remove onions and set aside. Dredge liver in flour seasoned with pepper. Melt 2 tablespoons margarine in pan and cook liver until done; put on hot platter. Pour off fat, add onion and vinegar to skillet. Heat and pour over liver. Sprinkle with parsley and serve. Makes 6 servings.

Each serving equals: **2 OUNCES MEAT**
                             1/2 VEGETABLE
                             1 SALTED FAT

POT ROAST OF BEEF

1-1/2 Pounds Round Steak
3 Tablespoons Margarine
1/2 Cup Diced Onions
1/4 Cup Diced Celery
1/4 Cup Diced Carrots
2-1/2 Tablespoons Flour
1 Cup Water

4 Tablespoons Tomato Paste
   (Canned Without Salt)
1 Bay Leaf
1/8 Teaspoon Thyme
1 Tablespoon Cornstarch
1/4 Cup Water

Heat 1 tablespoon margarine in skillet. Brown steak and remove to baking dish. Add remaining 2 tablespoons margarine to skillet. Add onions, celery and carrots, saute until tender, stirring frequently. Stir flour into mixture and cook several minutes, stirring frequently. Slowly add 1 cup water, stir and cook several minutes. Add tomato paste, bay leaf and thyme. Mix well. Mix cornstarch and 1/4 cup water and slowly add to hot vegetable mixture. Stir and cook till smooth and thick. Pour vegetable mixture over meat, cover and cook at 350° 2 hours or until tender. Slice meat and divide meat and vegetables into 8 equal servings.

Each serving equals: **2 OUNCES MEAT**
                               1 VEGETABLE

HOT ROAST BEEF SANDWICHES

Follow pot roast of beef recipe, when meat is cooked, slice into thin slices and serve over bread. Makes eight 1/2-cup servings of meat in gravy.

**Each 1/2 cup of meat
in gravy equals:**   **2 OUNCES MEAT**
                               1 VEGETABLE

SAUERBRATEN

1-3/4 Pounds Chuck Roast
1-1/2 Cups Water
1/2 Cup Distilled Vinegar
1/2 Cup Sliced Onions
Sugar Substitute to Equal
  2 Tablespoons Sugar
4 Peppercorns

1 Whole Clove
1 Bay Leaf
1/2 Sliced Lemon
1/4 Cup Margarine
2 Tablespoons Flour

Place meat in large bowl. Add water, vinegar, sliced onions, sugar substitute, peppercorns, whole clove, bay leaf and sliced lemon. Cover; marinate in refrigerator for at least 4 hours or several days. Turn meat several times.

Remove meat from marinade, drain thoroughly. Strain and reserve marinade. Melt 2 tablespoons margarine in skillet, brown meat. Add 1 cup marinade (reserve the rest). Cover and simmer 2-1/2 to 3 hours or until meat is tender. If necessary, add more marinade. Remove meat to warm platter. Pour off liquid from pan and set aside.

Melt 2 tablespoons margarine in saucepan, blend in flour, stirring constantly until mixture is golden brown. Remove from heat. Gradually add reserved cooking liquid, marinade and enough water to make 1-1/2 cups liquid. Return to heat, bring to a boil and cook, stirring constantly 1 to 2 minutes. Serve over meat. Makes 10 servings of meat and gravy.

Each serving equals: **2 OUNCES MEAT**

SHERRIED STROGANOFF

3 Tablespoons Margarine
1 Cup Sliced Onions
1-1/2 Cups Fresh, Sliced Mushrooms
6 Tablespoons Flour
1/4 Teaspoon Pepper
1 Pound Round Steak, Cut into Strips 1-1/2 Inches Long
1/2 Cup Sherry (Not Cooking Sherry)
1/4 Cup Water
3/4 Cup Sour Cream

Melt 1 tablespoon margarine in a large frying pan. Saute onions and mushrooms until tender. Remove vegetables and reserve. Add remaining margarine to frying pan. Toss beef strips in flour and pepper. Brown evenly in margarine, stirring often. Add sherry and water. Simmer covered for 45 minutes or until meat is tender. Mix in reserved vegetables. Slowly add sour cream, stir until smooth. Heat, but do not boil. Serve over noodles. Makes six 1/2-cup servings.

Each 1/2 cup serving equals:　　　2 OUNCES MEAT
　　　　　　　　　　　　　　　　　　　1/2 UNSALTED STARCH
　　　　　　　　　　　　　　　　　　　1 VEGETABLE
　　　　　　　　　　　　　　　　　　　1 SALTED FAT

SPAGHETTI SAUCE

1/8 Teaspoon Garlic Powder
1/4 Cup Minced Onion
1 Tablespoon Margarine
1-1/2 Pounds Ground Beef
One 1-Pound Can Low-Sodium Tomatoes
One 6-Ounce Can Tomato Paste (Canned Without Salt)
1 Tablespoon Sugar
1 Teaspoon Basil
1 Teaspoon Oregano
1 Teaspoon Pepper
Water

Saute garlic and onion in margarine. Add ground beef and brown thoroughly. Using a wooden spoon, smash canned tomatoes. Add tomatoes, tomato paste, sugar, basil, oregano and pepper to ground beef. Simmer 30 minutes. Add enough water to make 4 cups sauce. Makes eight 1/2-cup servings.

Each serving equals: **2 OUNCES MEAT**
2 VEGETABLES

STUFFED CABBAGE ROLLS

12 Cabbage Leaves
1 Pound Ground Beef
1/2 Cup Uncooked Long
   Grain Rice
1/4 Cup Grated Onion
2 Eggs, Beaten
1/4 Teaspoon Pepper
1/8 Teaspoon Allspice

2 Teaspoons Parsley
1/4 Cup Water
3 Ounces Tomato Paste
   (Canned Without Salt)
2 Tablespoons Lemon Juice
1 Cup Water
1/8 Teaspoon Pepper
1 Tablespoon Sugar

In large kettle, bring 3 quarts of water to a boil. Add cabbage, simmer 2 to 3 minutes, or until leaves are pliable. Remove cabbage and drain. Carefully remove 12 large leaves from cabbage, trim thick ribs. If inside leaves are not soft enough to roll, return to boiling water for a minute. In a large bowl, combine beef, rice, onion, eggs, pepper, allspice, parsley and 1/4 cup water. Mix together with a fork until well blended. Place about 1/4 cup meat mixture in hollow of each cabbage leaf. Fold sides of leaf over stuffing. Roll up from thick end of the leaf. Arrange rolls with seam side down in baking dish. Top with sauce made by combining tomato paste, lemon juice, 1 cup water and pepper. Bring cabbage rolls to boil over medium heat. Sprinkle with sugar; cover and bake at 375° for 1-1/2 hours. Uncover and bake 1-1/2 hours longer. Makes 6 servings, 2 cabbage rolls to a serving.

Each serving equals:　　　**2 OUNCES MEAT**
2 VEGETABLES

STUFFED FLANK STEAK

1-1/2 Pounds Flank Steak
2 Tablespoons Margarine
1/2 Cup Chopped Celery
2 Tablespoons Minced Onion
2-1/2 Cups Bread Cubes
1 Teaspoon Parsley
1/4 Teaspoon Poultry Seasoning
1/4 Teaspoon Marjoram

1/8 Teaspoon Pepper
2 Tablespoons Margarine
2 Cups Fresh Sliced Mushrooms
1 Tablespoon Margarine
1/4 Cup Red Wine
1-1/2 Tablespoons Flour
1 Cup Water

Wipe steak with damp paper towels. Score in diamond pattern 1/8-inch deep on both sides. Melt 2 tablespoons margarine in dutch oven. Add celery and onion, saute until tender; remove from heat. Add bread cubes, parsley, poultry seasoning, marjoram and pepper; toss lightly. Place stuffing lengthwise down the center of the steak, roll and secure with skewers or tie. Melt 2 tablespoons margarine in dutch oven and saute mushrooms until tender, remove mushrooms from pan. Melt 1 tablespoon margarine in the dutch oven, add the steak and brown well on all sides. Spoon mushrooms and wine over steak, cover and bake at 350° 1-1/2 hours until tender. Remove steak to warm platter. Mix flour and water, add to mushrooms and meat juices. Heat to boiling, stirring constantly. To serve, cut steak crosswise, pour gravy over steak. Makes 9 servings.

Each serving equals: **2 OUNCES MEAT**
                              1 VEGETABLE

STUFFED PEPPER CUPS

5 Medium Green Peppers (1 Pound)
1 Pound Ground Beef
1/2 Cup Chopped Onions
1/4 Teaspoon Pepper
One 1-Pound Can Low-Sodium Tomatoes
1/2 Cup Water
1/2 Cup Uncooked Long Grain Rice
1/4 Cup Dry Bread Crumbs

Cut peppers in half lengthwise, remove seeds and membrane. Precook in boiling water 5 minutes, drain. Cook ground beef and onions until meat is browned. Add pepper, tomatoes, water and rice. Cover and simmer until rice is tender, about 15 minutes. Stuff peppers with meat mixture, place in baking dish. Top with bread crumbs. Bake, uncovered, at 350° for 25 minutes. Makes 5 servings, 2 halves per serving.

Each serving equals:　　　**2 OUNCES MEAT**
　　　　　　　　　　　　　　　2 VEGETABLES
　　　　　　　　　　　　　　　1 UNSALTED STARCH

CHICKEN BREASTS AND MUSHROOMS IN WINE

2 Tablespoons Margarine
2 Whole, Split, Chicken Breasts
2 Green Onions
1/8 Teaspoon Pepper
1-1/2 Cups Sliced Fresh Mushrooms
1/3 Cup White Wine or Vermouth (Do Not Use Cooking Wine)

Melt the margarine in a skillet and brown the skin side of the chicken. Turn chicken over, add the onions and saute for 10 minutes, until chicken is golden and onions tender. Season with pepper. Add mushrooms and wine, scraping any bits that are stuck on the bottom of the pan. Cover and cook over low heat for 20 minutes or until chicken is tender. Remove the chicken, onions and mushrooms to a warm platter. Cook the pan juices over high heat, stirring a few minutes to reduce. Pour over chicken and serve. Divide into 8 servings.

Each serving equals: 2 OUNCES MEAT

CHICKEN CACCIATORE

2-1/2 Pounds Chicken Pieces
1/4 Cup Margarine
1/8 Teaspoon Garlic Powder
1/2 Teaspoon Italian Herbs

Cacciatore Sauce
(See Recipe Page H 4)

Brown chicken pieces in margarine and garlic powder. Sprinkle with Italian herbs, cover and simmer 40 to 50 minutes until tender. Prepare cacciatore sauce according to recipe. Serve hot sauce over chicken, accompanied by rice or noodles. Makes 5 servings.

Each serving equals: **2 OUNCES MEAT**
                               1 VEGETABLE
                               1 SALTED FAT

CHICKEN CROQUETTES

1/4 Cup Margarine
1/4 Cup Finely Chopped Onion
1/3 Cup Flour
1 Cup Milk
1 Cup Chopped Celery

2 Cups Chopped Cooked Chicken
1-1/3 Cup Dry Bread Crumbs
1 Egg
2 Tablespoons Water

Melt margarine in small saucepan, add onion and saute until tender. Stir in flour and add milk. Cook over medium high heat, stir constantly until mixture thickens. Remove from heat, add celery and chicken. Spread mixture in shallow dish and chill 2 hours. Place bread crumbs on waxed paper. Beat egg with water in small bowl. Cut chilled mixture into 7 equal portions. Using spoon, drop and roll each portion in crumbs. Shape into cones. Coat with egg mixture and roll in crumbs again. Refrigerate at least 2 hours or overnight. Heat oil to 375° in deep fat fryer. Fry croquettes until golden brown, about 2-3 minutes. Drain on paper towels, serve hot with hollandaise sauce (See Recipe, Page H 5). Makes 7 servings.

Each croquette equals:
2 OUNCES MEAT
1 SALTED STARCH
1 SALTED FAT

TURKEY CROQUETTES

Substitute 2 cups chopped, cooked turkey for chicken.

TUNA CROQUETTES

Substitute two 6-1/2-ounce cans of tuna, drained, for chicken.

CHICKEN PAPRIKASH

2-1/2 Pound Broiling Chicken, Cut Up
1/4 Teaspoon Pepper
1/8 Teaspoon Garlic Powder
2 Tablespoons Margarine
1 Cup Coarsley Chopped Onions
2 Medium Carrots, Thinly Sliced
1 Cup Water
1/2 Teaspoon Paprika
1 Cup Sour Cream
1 Teaspoon Parsley

Sprinkle chicken pieces with pepper and garlic powder. Brown a few pieces at a time in margarine in a large skillet. Remove chicken from skillet. Cook onions and carrots in same skillet for 5 minutes. Stir in water and paprika. Bring to a boil. Return chicken to pan. Cover and cook over low heat until chicken is tender, about 30 minutes. Transfer chicken to warm serving dish. Stir sour cream into sauce in skillet and heat, but do not boil. Pour sauce over chicken. Sprinkle with parsley. Makes 6 servings.

Each serving equals: **2 OUNCES MEAT**
                             1/2 VEGETABLE

CHICKEN WITH WINE AND GRAPES

1 Tablespoon Flour
1/4 Teaspoon Pepper
2-1/2 Pound Chicken, Cut Up
6 Tablespoons Margarine
1/4 Cup Dry White Wine (Do Not Use Cooking Wine)
1/2 Cup Water
1 Teaspoon Parsley
1 Tablespoon Honey
1/4 Teaspoon Pepper
1 Bay Leaf
2 Tablespoons Grated Orange Rind
1 Cup Halved White Grapes

Combine flour and 1/4 teaspoon pepper, use to lightly dust chicken parts. Melt margarine in large skillet. Add chicken and saute over medium heat, until golden brown on all sides. Add wine, water, parsley, honey, 1/4 teaspoon pepper and bay leaf. Cover, simmer over low heat 15 minutes. Add orange rind. Continue cooking until tender (10-15 minutes). Remove chicken to serving platter. Add grapes to gravy and cook, stirring constantly, 2 minutes. Pour over chicken, Serves 5.

Each serving equals: **2 OUNCES MEAT**
                                 1 FRUIT
                                 1 SALTED FAT

LEMON BROILED CHICKEN

1/2 Broiling Chicken, Cut-Up
1/4 Cup Lemon Juice
2 Tablespoons Oil
1/4 Teaspoon Thyme
1/4 Teaspoon Marjoram
1 Teaspoon Grated Lemon Rind

Arrange chicken in broiler pan. Combine remaining ingredients, brush on chicken. Broil 6 inches from heat for 1/2 hour on each side, baste frequently with the lemon mixture. Makes approximately 5 ounces.

Each ounce of chicken equals:

1 OUNCE MEAT

THE BASTING SAUCE IS FREE

RICE-STUFFED CHICKEN

3/4 Cup Uncooked Rice
6 Tablespoons Margarine
1/2 Cup Chopped Onion
1/2 Cup Chopped Green Pepper
1/2 Teaspoon Sage
1/4 Teaspoon Thyme
1/8 Teaspoon Pepper
4 Pound Roasting Chicken
2 Tablespoons Margarine

Cook rice according to package directions, omitting salt. Melt 6 tablespoons margarine in skillet. Add onion and green pepper and saute. Combine cooked rice, sauteed onion and green pepper, sage, thyme and pepper. Toss lightly with a fork. Stuff chicken with rice mixture. Rub 2 tablespoons margarine on chicken. Bake at 325° for 2 hours. Baste occasionally with pan juices. Makes six 1/2-cup servings of rice stuffing.

**Each serving of
rice stuffing equals:**   **1 UNSALTED STARCH
1 SALTED FAT**

**Each ounce of
chicken equals:**   **1 OUNCE MEAT**

CHICKEN 'N ORANGE SALAD

1 Cup Chopped, Cooked Chicken
1/2 Cup Diced Celery
1/2 Cup Green Pepper, Chopped

1/4 Cup Finely Sliced Onion
1 Cup Mandarin Oranges
1/3 Cup Mayonnaise

Toss chicken, celery, green pepper and onion to mix. Add mandarin oranges and mayonnaise. Mix gently. Makes three 1-cup servings.

Each serving equals: 2 OUNCES MEAT
                        1/2 FRUIT
                        1 SALTED FAT

HAWAIIAN CHICKEN SALAD

1/2 Cup Diced Celery
1-1/4 Cups Shredded Head Lettuce
1-1/2 Cups Chopped,
  Cooked Chicken
1 Cup Drained Unsweetened
  Pineapple Chunks
1/2 Teaspoon Sugar

2 Teaspoons Lemon Juice
1/2 Cup Mayonnaise
Dash "Tabasco" Sauce
1/4 Teaspoon Pepper
Paprika

Place celery, lettuce, chicken and pineapple in a bowl. Mix sugar, lemon juice, mayonnaise, "tabasco" and pepper together; add to chicken mixture and toss to mix. Serve on a lettuce leaf. Sprinkle with paprika. Makes four 3/4-cup servings.

Each serving equals: 2 OUNCES MEAT
                        1 FRUIT
                        1 SALTED FAT

CHOPPED CHICKEN LIVERS

1 Pound Chicken Livers
2 Tablespoons Margarine
1/2 Cup Chopped Onions
1 Medium Carrot, Thinly Sliced
2 Tablespoons Sherry (Do Not Use Cooking Sherry)
2 Tablespoons Margarine
3 Hard Cooked Eggs
1/4 Teaspoon Pepper
Dash Paprika
Dash Ground Ginger
Dash Oregano
2 Tablespoons Mayonnaise

Wash livers and remove any discolored spots, drain. Heat 2 tablespoons margarine in fry pan, add onions and carrots and brown. When browned, add several drops of water and let sizzle. Scrape pan. Remove onions and carrots. Add the livers, sherry and 2 tablespoons margarine to the pan and cook for 10 minutes or until browned. Grind or chop onions, livers and eggs until smooth and pasty. Add pepper, paprika, ginger, oregano and mayonnaise. Mix until creamy. Makes seven 1/2-cup servings.

Each serving equals: 2 OUNCES MEAT
                         1 SALTED FAT

TURKEY BROCCOLI AU GRATIN

One 10-Ounce Package Broccoli
2 Cups Chopped, Cooked Turkey
1/3 Cup Margarine
1/3 Cup Flour
2 Cups "Coffee Rich"
1/4 Teaspoon Pepper
1/4 Cup White Wine (Do Not Use Cooking Wine)
1/4 Cup Grated Regular Cheddar Cheese*

Cook broccoli in boiling water until tender, drain. Lightly butter casserole dish. Layer 1/2 broccoli, 1/2 turkey, 1/2 broccoli and 1/2 turkey. Melt margarine in small saucepan. Remove from heat, stir in flour and pepper. Slowly add "Coffee Rich", stirring until smooth. Return to heat, stir until thick and smooth. Cook several minutes. Add wine, blend and remove from heat. Pour over turkey and broccoli. Top with cheese. Bake at 350° for 30 minutes, until bubbly. Makes 6 servings.

Each serving equals: **2 OUNCES MEAT**
                             1 VEGETABLE
                             1 SALTED FAT

* Regular cheddar cheese does contain salt. It has been specially calculated into this recipe. Use only as directed.

TURKEY GLORY SANDWICH

6 Ounces Cooked Turkey, Sliced Thin
6 Slices Bread
3 Tablespoons Margarine
8 Ounces Cream Cheese, at Room Temperature
1 Cup "Coffee Rich"
1/2 Cup Grated Parmesan Cheese*
1/8 Teaspoon Garlic Powder
1/4 Teaspoon Paprika

Toast bread and spread with margarine. Place turkey on toast. In a small saucepan, gradually mix "Coffee Rich" into cream cheese. Cook over medium heat till mixture begins to boil. Remove from heat and stir in parmesan cheese and garlic powder. Pour over sandwiches. Sprinkle with paprika and serve. Makes 6 sandwiches.

Each sandwich equals: 2 OUNCES MEAT
1 SALTED STARCH
2 SALTED FATS

* Parmesan cheese does contain salt. It has been specially calculated into this recipe. Use it only as directed.

TURKEY NOODLE CASSEROLE

2 Tablespoons Margarine
1/4 Cup Chopped Onion
1/4 Cup Chopped Green Pepper
8 Ounces Cream Cheese
1-1/2 Cups "Coffee Rich"
1/4 Teaspoon Pepper

1/8 Teaspoon Garlic Powder
1/2 Cup Parmesan Cheese*
1 Cup Chopped, Cooked Turkey
2 Cup Cooked Noodles
1/4 Cup Dry Bread Crumbs
1/4 Teaspoon Paprika

Saute onion and green pepper in margarine till tender, remove vegetables from pan. Add cream cheese to pan and gradually mix in "Coffee Rich". Cook over medium heat just until boiling; remove from heat and add pepper, garlic powder and parmesan cheese. Stir in turkey and noodles, pour into 1-1/2-quart casserole dish. Sprinkle with bread crumbs and paprika. Bake at 350° for 15 minutes. Makes 6 servings.

Each serving equals: **2 OUNCES MEAT**
                       1-1/2 SALTED STARCHES

* Parmesan cheese does contain salt. It has been specially calculated into this recipe. Use only as directed.

CHICKEN NOODLE CASSEROLE

Follow recipe for turkey noodle casserole. Substitute 1 cup of chopped, cooked chicken in place of the turkey.

HUNGARIAN PORK CHOPS

1 Pound Trimmed Loin Pork Chops (Cut 3 to a Pound)
1 Tablespoon Oil
1/2 Cup Water
1 Teaspoon Paprika
1/2 Teaspoon Caraway Seed
1/2 Teaspoon Dill Weed
1/2 Teaspoon Onion Powder
1/8 Teaspoon Garlic Powder
2/3 Cup Sour Cream

Heat oil in frying pan, brown chops. Remove chops, drain off excess oil. Add 1/2 cup water, paprika, caraway seed, dill weed, onion powder and garlic powder to pan. Stir, scraping up browned bits from the bottom of the pan. Return pork chops to pan. Cover and cook on low heat for 1 hour or until chops are tender. Add more water if necessary. Remove pork chops to warm serving dish. Add sour cream to pan. Stir well and heat (do not boil). Serve sauce over chops. Makes 3 servings.

Each serving equals: **2 OUNCES MEAT**

PIZZA

DOUGH
  1 Package Dry Yeast
  1/4 Cup Lukewarm Water
  1/2 Teaspoon Sugar
  2-1/4 Cup Flour
  1/2 Cup Lukewarm Water
  1 Tablespoon Oil

In a small bowl dissolve yeast in 1/4 cup warm water with sugar. In a large bowl place 2 cups of flour; add yeast, 1/2 cup water and oil. Stir until mixture forms a soft dough. Knead dough on a surface floured with remaining 1/4 cup flour for 10 minutes until the dough is smooth and elastic. Transfer the dough to a large bowl, oiled lightly. Turn dough to coat with oil. Loosely cover with plastic wrap or a towel and let rise in a warm place for 1 hour or until double in bulk. Divide dough in half. Pat each half of the dough into a lightly greased pizza pan making a rim around the edge.

SAUCE
  One 6-Ounce Can Tomato Paste (Canned Without Salt)
  1/2 Cup Water
  1/4 Teaspoon Garlic Powder
  1 Tablespoon Oregano
  1 Tablespoon Basil
  1/4 Teaspoon Pepper
  2 Tablespoons Olive Oil (Optional)

Combine tomato paste, water, garlic powder, oregano, basil and pepper. Mix well. Spread half on each pizza crust. Sprinkle with olive oil, if desired.

PIZZA

TOPPINGS
 Italian Sausage (See Recipe Page E 35)
 1 Cup Sliced Fresh Mushrooms
 1/2 Cup Chopped Green Peppers
 1/2 Cup Chopped Onions
 8 Ounces Thinly Sliced or Grated Mozzarella Cheese*

Make sausage according to recipe using 1 pound ground pork. Cook, stirring, breaking up chunks until browned. Drain off fat. Spread evenly using half for each pizza. Divide mushrooms, green peppers and onions between pizzas and top with cheese. Bake at 425° for 15 minutes. Makes 2 pizzas. Cut each into 8 slices. Pizza may be frozen before cooking, cooked pizza is also good reheated.

Two slices equal:
 2 OUNCES MEAT
 2 UNSALTED STARCHES
 1 VEGETABLE
 1 SALTED FAT

Three slices equal:
 3 OUNCES MEAT
 2-1/2 UNSALTED STARCHES
 1-1/2 VEGETABLES
 1 SALTED FAT

* Mozzarella cheese does contain added salt. It has been specially calculated into this recipe. Use only as directed.

ROAST PORK
WITH APPLES AND RAISINS

2-1/2 Pound Boneless Pork Roast (Tenderloin or Loin)
1/8 Teaspoon Pepper
1/8 Teaspoon Nutmeg
1/8 Teaspoon Allspice

SAUCE
  2/3 Cup Apple Juice
  1/2 Cup Raisins
  1-1/4 Teaspoons Cinnamon
  1/2 Cup Pork Drippings
  2 Cups Peeled, Cored and Diced Apples
  2 Teaspoons Cornstarch
  1/3 Cup Apple Juice

Rub roast with pepper, nutmeg and allspice. Place in baking pan and bake at 350° for 2-1/4 to 2-1/2 hours. Remove from oven and drain off pork drippings for sauce. Put roast back in oven to keep warm while preparing sauce.

Heat 2/3 cup apple juice in saucepan until warm. Add raisins, cinnamon, pork drippings and apples. Bring to a boil, stirring frequently. Mix cornstarch with 1/3 cup apple juice. Slowly add to the boiling apple and raisin mixture, stirring constantly while heating until thickened and smooth. Simmer for 5 minutes. Serve warm sauce over sliced meat. Makes 2-1/4 cups sauce and 24 ounces meat. Divide into 12 servings.

Each serving equals: **2 OUNCES MEAT**
                              1 FRUIT

SAUSAGE

1 Pound Lean Ground Pork
Desired Seasonings (See Recipes Below)

Mix seasonings thoroughly into ground pork. Refrigerate overnight. Make into 9 patties. Pan fry, bake or broil until done. Freeze uncooked patties individually until needed.

Each pattie equals: 1 OUNCE MEAT

ITALIAN SAUSAGE

1/4 Teaspoon Pepper
1/4 to 1/2 Teaspoon Crushed Red Pepper
3/4 Teaspoon Fennel

SPANISH SAUSAGE

1/8 to 1/4 Teaspoon
   Crushed Red Pepper
1/4 Teaspoon Garlic Powder
1/2 to 1 Tablespoon Chili Powder

1/8 Teaspoon Ground Cumin
1/2 to 1 Teaspoon Pepper
2 Tablespoons Vinegar

OLD-TIME COUNTRY SAUSAGE

1/2 Teaspoon Sage
1/8 Teaspoon Crushed Red Pepper
1/2 Teaspoon Pepper

NOTE: Use the lesser amounts of seasonings for milder sausage
         and the full amount for HOT sausage.

BREADED VEAL CUTLETS

1/2 Teaspoon Paprika
1 Pound Thin Veal Cutlets (6 Pieces)
1 Cup Fine Dry Bread Crumbs, Unseasoned
1-1/2 Teaspoons Parsley
2 Eggs, Beaten
1/4 Cup Margarine
1/4 Cup Oil
Lemon Slices

Sprinkle cutlets with paprika. Pound cutlets with mallet to flatten. Combine bread crumbs with parsley. Dip cutlets into eggs then coat with bread crumbs. Place on wire rack to dry for 15 minutes. Fry in mixture of margarine and oil at 375° for 3 to 4 minutes on each side or until done. Drain on paper towels. Garnish with lemon slices. Makes 6 servings.

Each serving equals: **2 OUNCES MEAT
1 SALTED STARCH**

OSSO BUCCO

1/4 Cup Margarine
Dash Garlic Powder
2 Tablespoons Finely Minced Onion
1 Pound Sliced Veal Shanks
1-1/2 Tablespoons Flour
Dash Pepper
1/4 Cup Water
1/4 Cup White Wine
2 Tablespoons Tomato Paste (Canned Without Salt)
1-1/2 Teaspoons Parsley
1 Teaspoon Grated Lemon Rind

Melt margarine in heavy skillet, and garlic powder and onion. Saute onion until tender. Dredge veal shanks in flour and pepper, brown in margarine and onions on both sides. Add water, wine and tomato paste. Cover tightly and simmer slowly 1-1/2 hours until tender, adding more water if necessary. Sprinkle with parsley and lemon rind before serving. Makes approximately 4 serving, 2 ounces of meat each.

**Each 2-ounce portion
of meat and 1/4
of the sauce equals:**   **2 OUNCES MEAT
1 VEGETABLE
1 SALTED FAT**

VEAL GOULASH

1/4 Cup Margarine
1 Pound Boneless Veal Cubes
3/4 Cup Chopped Onion
2 Teaspoons Paprika
2 Tablespoons Flour
1/4 Teaspoon Caraway Seeds
1 Bay Leaf
1/2 Teaspoon Parsley

1/8 Teaspoon Pepper
1-3/4 Cup Water
2 Tablespoons Tomato Paste
  (Canned Without Salt)
1 Tablespoon Cornstarch
1/4 Cup Water
1/2 Cup Sour Cream

Melt margarine in heavy skillet, add veal cubes and brown on all sides. Add onions and cook until transparent. Add paprika and flour. Stir and cook for 5 minutes. Add caraway seeds, bay leaf, parsley, pepper and 1-3/4 cup water. Bring to a boil. Cover and reduce heat, simmer slowly for 1 hour or until meat is tender. Mix tomato paste and cornstarch with 1/4 cup water. Add slowly, stirring constantly until sauce is thick and smooth. Slowly add sour cream, stirring constantly, do not allow to boil. Serve over noodles or rice. Makes six 1/2-cup portions.

Each serving equals: 2 OUNCES MEAT
                           1 VEGETABLE
                           1 SALTED FAT

VEAL PICCATTA

2 Veal Shoulder Chops
1 Tablespoon Flour
2 Tablespoons Margarine
1 Tablespoon Lemon Juice
Dash Pepper
1/4 Teaspoon Parsley

Remove veal from bone, trim fat. Pound meat with a meat cleaver until the chops are as thin as possible. Coat chops with flour. Melt margarine and brown chops lightly on both sides. Sprinkle with lemon juice. Season with pepper and parsley. Serve with lemon wedges. Makes approximately three 2-ounce servings.

Two ounces equal: **2 OUNCES MEAT**

VEAL WITH SOUR CREAM

1/2 Cup Diced Onion
1/4 Cup Margarine
1 Pound Veal, Cut Into 1-Inch Cubes
1 Cup White Wine
1/8 Teaspoon Garlic Powder
2 Teaspoons Basil
1/4 Teaspoon Pepper
1-1/2 Cups Sour Cream

In a heavy skillet, saute onion in margarine until soft. Add veal cubes and brown on all sides. Add wine, garlic powder, basil and pepper. Simmer gently, covered, for 15 minutes or until the veal is tender. Add sour cream and cook slowly, stirring until sauce is blended and thickened, do not boil. Serve over rice. Makes six 1/2-cup servings.

Each serving equals: **2 OUNCES MEAT**
                             1 VEGETABLE
                             1 SALTED FAT

LAMB CURRY

1/4 Cup Margarine
2 Cups Chopped Onions
1/8 Teaspoon Garlic Powder
1 Pound Boneless Lamb Shoulder, Cut Into 2-Inch Cubes
One 8-Ounce Container Plain Yogurt
1 Teaspoon Ginger
2 Teaspoons Coriander
1/4 Teaspoon Cinnamon
1/2 Teaspoon Cardamon
1/4 Teaspoon Ground Cloves

Melt margarine in heavy pan, add onions and garlic powder. Saute until onions are tender and transparent, remove from pan. Add the lamb to pan and brown on all sides. Return the onions to the pan and add yogurt, ginger, coriander, cinnamon, cardamon and cloves. Simmer until tender, about 30 minutes. If desired, thin sauce with water before serving. Serve over rice. Makes five 1/3-cup servings.

Each serving equals: **2 OUNCES MEAT**
                             1 VEGETABLE
                             1 SALTED FAT

SHISH KABOBS

1/4 Cup Minced Onion
2 Teaspoons Parsley
1/2 Teaspoon Marjoram
1/2 Teaspoon Thyme
1/4 Teaspoon Pepper
1/8 Teaspoon Garlic Powder
2 Tablespoons Lemon Juice
1 Pound Lean, Boneless Lamb,
  Cut Into 1-Inch Cubes

1 Green Pepper, Cut Into
  1-Inch Squares
1 Medium Tomato, Cut Into Chunks
2 Cups Small Whole Onions,
  Partially Cooked
1 Tablespoon Margarine, Melted

Combine onion, parsley, marjoram, thyme, pepper, garlic powder and lemon juice. Add meat, stir to coat. Refrigerate several hours or overnight, stirring occasionally. Alternate meat cubes and vegetables equally on 5 skewers. Place on broiler rack. Lightly brush vegetables with melted margarine. Spread on any remaining marinade mixture. Broil, about 4 inches from source of heat, turning once, until lamb and vegetables are tender and done, about 7 minutes per side. Makes 5 servings.

Each serving equals: **2 OUNCES MEAT**
                               1-1/2 VEGETABLES

BAKED CRAB IMPERIAL

1/4 Cup Margarine
1/4 Cup Flour
2 Cups Milk
1/8 Teaspoon Pepper
1/2 Teaspoon Celery Flakes
Dash Cayenne
1 Egg Yolk, Beaten
2 Tablespoons Sherry
1 Cup Soft Bread Crumbs
1 Pound Flaked Crab
1 Teaspoon Parsley
1 Teaspoon Minced Onion
1/4 Cup Dry Bread Crumbs
1/2 Teaspoon Paprika

Melt margarine, remove from heat. Stir in flour. Gradually stir in milk; add pepper, celery flakes and cayenne. Stir and cook until thick. Add a small amount of white sauce to egg yolk and mix. Add egg yolk back to white sauce, cook 2 minutes. Remove from heat and gently stir in sherry, soft bread crumbs, crab, parsley and onion. Pour into casserole, top with bread crumbs and paprika. Bake at 400° for 20 to 25 minutes. Makes six 1/2-cup servings.

Each serving equals: **2 OUNCES MEAT**
                            1 MILK
                            1/2 SALTED STARCH
                            1 SALTED FAT

COQUILLES ST. JACQUES

1/2 Pound Raw Scallops
1 Tablespoon Margarine
2 Green Onions, Chopped
1/2 Teaspoon Parsley
1 Stalk Celery
1/8 Teaspoon Thyme
1 Bay Leaf
1/2 Cup White Wine
  (Not cooking wine)
1 Tablespoon Margarine

1/2 Cup Fresh Sliced Mushrooms
2 Tablespoons Water
1 Tablespoon Lemon Juice
1/8 Teaspoon Pepper
1-1/2 Tablespoon Flour
1-1/2 Tablespoon Margarine
1 Egg Yolk
1/3 Cup Heavy Cream
2 Tablespoons Parmesan Cheese
2 Tablespoons Bread Crumbs

Dry scallops on paper towels. Place in a saucepan with 1 tablespoon margarine, green onions, a boquet garni (a cheesecloth bag) of parsley, celery, thyme and bay leaf. Barely cover with wine. Bring to a boil and simmer very gently for 4 or 5 minutes, or until scallops are just tender. Drain and save the broth, discard boquet garni. If large, cut the scallops in smaller pieces and set aside. Melt 1 tablespoon margarine in the saucepan, saute the mushrooms in it for a minute. Add water, lemon juice and pepper. Simmer mushrooms gently for a few minutes, then drain, combining the mushroom liquid with the reserved liquid from the scallops. Knead the flour with 1-1/2 tablespoons margarine, working them together into small balls the size of peas. Heat the reserved liquid from the scallops and mushrooms and gradually stir in the flour-margarine balls, one at a time. Cook and stir until the sauce is thickened and smooth, then cook for 2 to 3 minutes more. Add scallops and heat through. Beat the egg yolk with the cream, add the cream mixture to the sauce and cook gently, stirring until the sauce is very thick and smooth. Do not boil. Add the mushrooms. Spoon mixture into shells or individual dishes. Sprinkle with parmesan cheese and crumbs. Brown lightly under broiler and serve. Makes 3 servings.

Each serving equals: **2 OUNCES MEAT**
                            2 VEGETABLES
                            2 SALTED FATS

BROILED FISH

Arrange fish fillets in greased shallow baking pan. Brush lightly with melted margarine. Season with pepper, basil, garlic powder and a generous dusting of paprika. Broil 5 to 6 inches from heat until done through and golden. Allow 8 to 10 minutes for thin fillets and up to 15 minutes for thick. Serve with lemon wedges.

**Each ounce of
cooked fish equals:**   **1 OUNCE MEAT**

CRAB RICE CASSEROLE

12 Ounces Salt-Free, Cooked Crab
3 Cups Hot Cooked Rice
1 Cup Shredded Cheddar Cheese*
One 3-Ounce Package Cream Cheese, at Room Temperature
1 Cup Sour Cream
1/2 Cup Chopped Onion
1/8 Teaspoon Garlic Powder
1/2 Teaspoon Basil
1 Medium Tomato, Sliced

Combine crab, rice and cheddar cheese. Spoon half of the mixture into a shallow 1-1/2-quart baking dish. Beat cream cheese until smooth. Stir in sour cream, onion, garlic powder and basil; spoon half over crab mixture. Layer with remaining crab mixture and top with sour cream mixture. Cover dish with foil, crimping the edges. Bake at 350° for 30 minutes. Uncover and top with tomato slices. Return to oven for 5 minutes. Makes 6 servings.

Each serving equals: **2 OUNCES MEAT**
1 SALTED STARCH
1 SALTED FAT

* Cheddar cheese does contain salt. It has been specially calculated into this recipe. Use it only as directed.

FISH AU GRATIN

1 Pound Fresh or Frozen Unsalted Flounder, Sole or Haddock
1/3 Cup Mayonnaise
1/4 Cup Parmesan Cheese*
2 Tablespoons Dry Bread Crumbs

Brush each fish fillet with mayonnaise. Mix cheese and crumbs. Roll fish in crumb mixture, place in baking dish. Sprinkle with remaining crumb mixture. Bake at 375° until fish is lightly browned and flakes easily, 30 to 35 minutes for frozen fish or 25 minutes for thawed or fresh fish. Makes 5 servings.

Each serving equals: **2 OUNCES MEAT**
                                   1 SALTED FAT

*Parmesan cheese does contain some salt. It has been specially calculated into this recipe. Use only as directed.

HAWAIIAN SHRIMP SALAD

1 Cup Diced Celery
2 Cups Shredded Lettuce
1 Pound Raw Shrimp, Cooked
2 Cups Drained, Unsweetened Pineapple Chunks
3/4 Cup Mayonnaise
2 Teaspoons Pineapple Juice
Dash "Tabasco" Sauce

Combine celery, shredded lettuce, shrimp and pineapple chunks. Mix mayonnaise, pineapple juice, and "Tabasco"; add to shrimp mixture and toss to mix. Makes five 3/4-cup servings.

Each serving equals: **2 OUNCES MEAT**
                              1 FRUIT
                              2 SALTED FATS

SALMON PATTIES

Two 7-3/4 Ounce Cans Low-Sodium Salmon, Drained
2 Eggs
2 Tablespoons Diced Onions
8 Squares Low-Sodium Crackers, Crushed
Dash Pepper
Dash "Tabasco" Sauce

Flake salmon. Add remaining ingredients. Form into 6 patties. Fry lightly on both sides in margarine or bake on a lightly greased cookie sheet at 350° for 15 minutes. Makes 6 patties.

Each pattie equals: **2 OUNCES MEAT**

SEAFOOD QUICHE

1-Crust Pie Shell (See Recipe Page D 1)
1/2 Cup Chopped Onion
1/4 Cup Chopped Green Pepper
1-1/2 Cups Sliced Fresh Mushrooms
2 Tablespoons Margarine
1/2 Cup Salt-Free Cooked Shrimp, Crab, or Tuna
1-1/2 Cups Shredded Swiss Cheese*
3 Eggs
1 Cup "Coffee Rich"
Dash "Tabasco" Sauce

Prepare pie crust as directed and place in 9-inch pie pan and set aside. Saute onion, green pepper and mushrooms in margarine until tender. Dice shrimp or flake crab or tuna and place in pie shell. Combine cheese, eggs, "Coffee Rich", "Tabasco" and sauteed vegetables; mix thoroughly and pour into pie shell. Bake at 350° for 50 to 60 minutes until brown on top. Serve immediately. Makes 6 servings.

Each serving equals: 2 OUNCES MEAT
1-1/2 SALTED STARCHES
2 SALTED FATS

* Swiss cheese does contain salt. It has been specially calculated into this recipe. Use only as directed.

SHRIMP AND FISH CREOLE

1 Cup Uncooked Long Grain Rice
One 7-Ounce Package Frozen Shrimp
1/2 Pound Frozen Cod
1-1/2 Cups Chopped Onion
1/2 Cup Chopped Green Pepper
1/4 Teaspoon Garlic Powder
1 Tablespoon Margarine
One 1-Pound Can Low-Sodium Tomatoes, Undrained
1 Tablespoon Parsley
2 Teaspoons Paprika
1/2 Teaspoon Sugar
1/8 Teaspoon Cayenne Pepper
1 Bay Leaf
1 Tablespoon Cornstarch
1 Tablespoon Water

Cook rice according to package directions, omitting salt. Partially thaw shrimp and fish. Saute onions, green pepper, and garlic in margarine until tender, about 5 minutes. Chop tomatoes and add with parsley, paprika, sugar, cayenne and bay leaf. Cover and simmer 30 minutes. Cut cod into 1-inch squares. Add to sauce with shrimp. Cook about 5 minutes, stirring occasionally, until the shrimp turns pink and the fish flakes easily with a fork. Mix cornstarch and water. Add to creole and cook, stirring constantly, until slightly thickened. Serve creole over cooked rice. Makes five scant 3/4-cup servings creole over 1/3 cup rice.

Each serving equals: **2 OUNCES MEAT**
                             2 VEGETABLES
                             1-1/2 UNSALTED STARCHES

SHRIMP BROILED WITH GARLIC BUTTER

1 Pound Uncooked Shrimp
1/2 Cup Margarine
2 Teaspoons Lemon Juice
2 Tablespoons Minced Onions
1 Teaspoon Minced Garlic or 1/4 Teaspoon Garlic Powder
Dash Pepper
1 Tablespoon Parsley

Wash and dry shrimp. Melt margarine and add lemon juice, onions, garlic and pepper. Broil shrimp in garlic sauce 4 to 5 inches from heat for 5 minutes, turn and broil 5 more minutes. Serve on platter with strained pan juices. Sprinkle with parsley. Makes 5 servings.

Each serving equals: **2 OUNCES MEAT**
                               1 SALTED FAT

TUNA NOODLE CASSEROLE

Follow the recipe for turkey noodle casserole, Page E 30, substituting one 6-1/2-ounce can of low-sodium tuna for 1 cup of turkey. Makes 6 servings.

Each serving equals: **2 OUNCES MEAT**
1-1/2 UNSALTED STARCHES

TUNA RICE CASSEROLE

Substitute one 6-1/2-ounce can low-sodium canned tuna for crab in crab rice casserole recipe, Page E 46. Makes 6 servings.

Each serving equals: **2 OUNCES MEAT**
1 SALTED STARCH

TUNA PATTIES

Two 6-1/2-Ounce Cans Low-Sodium Tuna, Drained
2 Eggs
2 Tablespoons Diced Onions
8 Squares Low-Sodium Crackers, Crushed
Dash Pepper
Dash "Tabasco" Sauce

Flake tuna, add remaining ingredients. Form into 8 patties. Fry lightly on both sides in margarine or bake on a lightly greased cookie sheet at 350° for 15 minutes. Makes 8 patties.

Each pattie equals: 2 OUNCES MEAT

TUNA MACARONI SALAD

See recipe page G 5.

VEGETABLE FISH BAKE

1-1/2 Cups Sliced Onions
2 Tablespoons Margarine
1 Pound Fillet of Sole
1/4 Teaspoon Pepper
1/2 Cup Sliced Fresh Mushrooms
1 Green Pepper, Sliced
1/4 Cup White Wine (Not Cooking Wine)
1 Tablespoon Lemon Juice

Arrange onions on bottom of 9-inch square baking dish. Dot with margarine. Season both sides of fish with pepper. Place on top of onions. Top with mushrooms and green peppers. Combine wine and lemon juice, pour over vegetables. Bake at 350° until fish flakes easily, about 25 to 30 minutes. Makes six 2/3-cup servings.

Each serving equals: **2 OUNCES MEAT**
                            1 VEGETABLE

EGG SALAD

1 Hard Boiled Egg
2 Tablespoons Mayonnaise
2 Teaspoons Diced Low-Sodium Pickles
Dash Pepper

Dice egg; add mayonnaise, pickles and pepper, mix lightly. Serve on lettuce, in a sandwich, or in a grilled sandwich.

Each serving equals: **1 OUNCE MEAT**
                               1 SALTED FAT

MEAT SALADS

2 Ounces Low-Sodium Salmon, Tuna, Chicken or Turkey, Diced
2 Tablespoons Mayonnaise
2 Teaspoons Diced Low-Sodium Pickles, if desired
Dash Pepper

Combine meat with mayonnaise, pickles and pepper. Serve on lettuce leaf, in a sandwich or in a grilled sandwich.

Each serving equals: **2 OUNCES MEAT**
                               1 SALTED FAT

SCRAMBLED POTATOES
AND EGGS

2 Tablespoons Margarine
1 Cup Cold, Left Over, Specially Prepared Potatoes*
Dash Pepper
6 Eggs
1/2 Cup Light Cream
1/8 Teaspoon Pepper

Melt margarine in small skillet. Brown potatoes lightly in margarine. Sprinkle with pepper. Beat eggs, cream and 1/8 teaspoon pepper together lightly. Pour over potatoes. Stir until eggs are done. Makes 3 servings.

Each serving equals: **2 OUNCES MEAT**
                             1 UNSALTED STARCH (POTATO)
                             1 SALTED FAT

* To make specially prepared potatoes, peel and slice potatoes into 1/8-inch slices. Soak in a large amount of water (5 cups for every cup of potatoes) 2 hours or overnight. Drain and cook in large amount of water (5 cups for every cup of potatoes) until tender. Drain and serve as desired.

Limit to 1 Serving of Potato a Day.

FETTUCCINI ALFREDO

One 6-Ounce Package Fettuccini or Egg Noodles
1/2 Cup Light Whipping Cream
2 Tablespoons Margarine, Softened
Dash Pepper
1/2 Cup Grated Parmesan Cheese*

Cook noodles as directed on package, omitting salt. Drain well. Transfer to serving dish. Beat whipping cream, margarine and pepper until thick and creamy. Do not overbeat. Add parmesan cheese; pour over hot noodles and toss until evenly covered. Serve immediately. Makes four 1-cup servings.

Each serving equals: **1 OUNCE MEAT**
                                 2 UNSALTED STARCHES
                                 1 SALTED FAT

* Parmesan cheese does contain salt. It has been specially calculated into this recipe. Use only as directed.

MACARONI AND CHEESE

2 Cup Uncooked Elbow Macaroni
1/4 Cup Margarine
1/4 Cup Flour
1/8 Teaspoon Pepper
2 Cups Milk
8 Ounces (2 Cups) Grated Cheddar Cheese*

Cook macaroni in unsalted water until macaroni is cooked but firm. Drain and set aside. Melt margarine in saucepan, remove from heat, stir in flour and pepper. Gradually stir in milk. Stir until smooth, return to heat and continue to cook and stir until slightly thickened. Add 3/4 of the grated cheese. Combine with macaroni. Place mixture in 2-quart casserole and sprinkle evenly with remaining cheese. Bake uncovered at 350° for 30 minutes. Makes six 3/4-cup servings.

Each serving equals: 1-1/2 OUNCES MEAT
2 SALTED STARCHES
1 SALTED FAT

* Regular cheese does contain salt. It has been specially calculated into this recipe. Use only as directed.

MEAT COATINGS

BASIC MIX
  1 Cup Dry Unseasoned Breadcrumbs
  1/4 Teaspoon Pepper
  1/2 Teaspoon Garlic Powder
  1/2 Teaspoon Basil
  1/2 Teaspoon Dried Celery Leaves
  1/2 Teaspoon Paprika

Blend in blender or food processor until fine. To use, dip meat in melted margarine and coat with crumbs, one piece at a time. Place meat in a pan and bake until done.

BEEF OR VEAL CUTLETS

Add 1/2 teaspoon marjoram or oregano to basic mix. Coat meat with melted margarine, then coat with mix, bake at 300° for 1 hour. Mix recipe is sufficient for 6 to 8 cutlets.

CHICKEN

Add 1/2 teaspoon thyme and 1/2 teaspoon sage to basic mix. Dip chicken pieces in melted margarine and coat chicken pieces with mix. Bake at 350° for 50 minutes. Mix recipe is sufficient for 1 cut-up chicken. Makes a wonderful oven-fried chicken.

PORK CHOPS

Add 1/2 teaspoon dried tarragon or 1/4 teaspoon allspice to basic mix. Coat chops with melted margarine, then with mix. Bake at 350° for 45 minutes. Mix recipe is sufficient for 6 pork chops.

1/6 of meat coating
recipes equals:　　　　**1 SALTED STARCH**

VEGETABLES

DILLED GREEN BEANS

One 10-Ounce Package Frozen Green Beans
1/2 Cup Thinly Sliced Onion
2 Tablespoons Margarine
2 Teaspoons Dried Dill Weed
1/8 Teaspoon Pepper
1 Teaspoon Lemon Peel

Cook green beans and onion in boiling water until beans are tender, about 20 minutes. Drain. Stir in margarine, dill, pepper and lemon peel. Makes 3 servings.

Each serving equals: **1 VEGETABLE**
                             1/2 SALTED FAT

CURRIED CORN

One 10-Ounce Package Frozen Corn
2 Tablespoons Margarine
3/4 Teaspoon Curry Powder

Cook corn and drain. Add margarine and curry powder. Stir until margarine is melted and curry powder is thoroughly mixed. Makes four scant 1/2-cup servings.

Each serving equals: **1 VEGETABLE**
                             1 SALTED FAT

GOURMET GREEN BEANS

One 10-Ounce Package Frozen Green Beans
1-1/2 Tablespoons Margarine
1 Teaspoon Lemon Juice
1 Teaspoon Parsley
Dash Pepper

Cook green beans in large amount of boiling water for 15 minutes. Drain, add margarine, lemon juice, parsley and pepper. Toss green beans to coat well. Makes 3 servings.

Each serving equals:　　**1 VEGETABLE**
　　　　　　　　　　　　　1/2 SALTED FAT

GREEN BEANS AND MUSHROOMS

Make gourmet green beans (above) omitting parsley. Saute 1 cup fresh sliced mushrooms in 1 tablespoon margarine and add to hot seasoned green beans. Makes 4 servings.

Each serving equals:　　**1 VEGETABLE**
　　　　　　　　　　　　　1/2 SALTED FAT

SAVORY BRUSSELS SPROUTS

2 Cups Brussels Sprouts
1/4 Cup Margarine
1/4 Teaspoon Pepper
1/2 Teaspoon Lemon Juice

Trim brussels sprouts. Cook in large amount of boiling water for 5 minutes; drain. Add margarine, cook and shake well for 3 to 4 minutes to coat well. Add pepper and lemon juice. Makes six 1/4-cup servings.

Each serving equals: **1 VEGETABLE**
                              1/2 SALTED FAT

HARVARD BEETS

1 Pound Can Low-Sodium Beets   **1/3 Cup Water**
Sugar Substitute to Equal   **1/4 Cup Vinegar**
** 2 Tablespoons Sugar**   **2 Tablespoons Margarine**
1 Tablespoon Cornstarch

Drain beets. In saucepan, combine sugar substitute and cornstarch. Stir in water, vinegar and margarine. Cook and stir until mixture thickens and bubbles. Add beets, heat through. Makes 4 servings.

Each serving equals: **1 VEGETABLE**
                              1 SALTED FAT

FRIED CABBAGE AND NOODLES

1-1/2 Cups Cabbage (About 1/8 Head Raw)
1/2 Cup Dry Noodles
2 Tablespoons Margarine
1/4 Teaspoon Onion Powder
1/4 to 1/2 Teaspoon Caraway Seeds

Separate the cabbage leaves, rinse to clean. Soak in large amount of warm water for 2 hours; drain. Boil in large amount of water for 15 minutes; drain. Cook noodles in unsalted boiling water until tender; drain. Dice the cabbage into fairly small pieces. Melt margarine in a large frying pan. Add cooked cabbage and onion powder. Fry, until cabbage begins to brown slightly (about 15 minutes). Add the noodles and caraway seeds. Heat thoroughly and serve. Makes five 1/2-cup servings.

Each serving equals: 1/2 SALTED STARCH

LEMON CARROTS

3 Cups Cooked Sliced Carrots
Sugar Substitute to Equal 1 Tablespoon Sugar
2 Tablespoons Margarine
1 Tablespoon Lemon Juice
1/4 Teaspoon Grated Lemon Peel

Cook carrots in large amount of water until just tender, drain well. Add sugar substitute, margarine, lemon juice and lemon peel. Heat and stir until margarine is melted. Makes six 1/2-cup servings.

Each serving equals: 1 VEGETABLE

CARROTS VICHY

2 Cups Sliced Carrots   **1/8 Teaspoon Marjoram**
2 Tablespoons Margarine   **1 Teaspoon Parsley**
1/4 Teaspoon Sugar

Cook carrots until just tender in large amount of water, drain. Add margarine and shake to coat well. Add sugar and marjoram, sprinkle with parsley. Makes four 1/2-cup servings.

Each serving equals: 1 VEGETABLE
**   1/2 SALTED FAT**

HOT DEVILED CARROTS

2 Tablespoons Margarine
2 Cups Cooked Sliced Carrots
Sugar Substitute to Equal 1-1/2 Tablespoons Sugar
1 Teaspoon Dry Mustard
Dash "Tabasco" Sauce
Dash Pepper

Melt margarine in saucepan; add carrots and cook 3 minutes over low heat, until coated with margarine. Add sugar substitute, mustard, "Tabasco" and pepper; mix well. Cover and cook over low heat for 5 minutes, stirring frequently. Makes four 1/2-cup servings.

Each serving equals: **1 VEGETABLE**
                              1/2 SALTED FAT

HOT CABBAGE SLAW

Sugar Substitute to Equal
  2 Tablespoons Sugar
1 Tablespoon Minced Onion
1/2 Teaspoon Caraway Seed
1/2 Teapoon Dry Mustard
1/4 Teaspoon Pepper

3 Tablespoons Vinegar
2 Tablespoons Margarine
4 Cups Finely Shredded
  Cabbage
1 Cup Unpeeled Diced Apple

Combine substitute sugar, onion, caraway seed, dry mustard, pepper and vinegar. Blend thoroughly and set aside. In a large skillet melt margarine. Add cabbage and apple, saute over medium heat for 3 minutes. Stir in vinegar mixture and simmer on low heat stirring occasionally, until apples and cabbage are tender, (about 5 minutes.) Makes 6 servings.

Each serving equals: **1 VEGETABLE**

FRIED POTATOES

4 Cups Specially Prepared Potatoes
1/3 Cup Margarine
1/2 Cup Chopped Onions
1/2 Cup Chopped Green Pepper
1/2 Teaspoon Pepper
1/4 Teaspoon Paprika
1 Tablespoon Parsley

Peel and slice potatoes in thin slices (1/8-inch thick) and soak in 5 quarts of water at least 2 hours or overnight. Drain well. Cook in 5 quarts of boiling water until just tender, drain well. Melt margarine in a large skillet. Add potatoes, onion and green pepper. Sprinkle with pepper and paprika. Cook, uncovered, over medium heat, about 20 minutes. Sprinkle with parsley just before serving. Makes six 1/2-cup servings.

Each serving equals: 1 UNSALTED STARCH (POTATO)
**   1 SALTED FAT**

Limit to 1 Serving Potato a Day.

OVEN FRIED POTATOES

FOR EACH SERVING:
  1 Medium Potato
  1 Tablespoon Oil

OPTIONAL SEASONING:
  Dust with Paprika
  Pinch of Cayenne
  Pinch of Garlic Powder
  Pinch of Onion Powder

Peel potatoes and cut into french-fry strips. Soak at least 2 hours in a large pan of water (at least 5 cups water for 1 cup of potatoes). Drain and pat dry with paper towels. Measure 1 tablespoon oil into a bowl for each potato. Add potatoes and toss with a spoon, coating them lightly but thoroughly with oil. Spread the potatoes on a cookie sheet, not touching, and bake at 425° for 10 minutes, or until brown. Reduce heat to 350° and bake another 20 to 30 minutes, turning occasionally, until done through. Serve immediately, dust with seasonings if desired. Each potato makes one serving.

Each serving equals: 1 UNSALTED STARCH (POTATO)

Limit to 1 Serving Potato a Day.

POTATO PANCAKES

4 Large Potatoes, Pared
1/4 Cup Grated Onion
2 Eggs, Slightly Beaten
2 Tablespoons Flour
Dash Nutmeg
Dash Pepper
Oil for Frying

On a medium grater, grate potatoes. Drain well. Measure 3 cups of potatoes. Soak grated potatoes in 4 quarts of water at least 2 hours. Drain very well, pat dry with paper towels.

In a large bowl, combine potatoes, onion, eggs, flour, nutmeg and pepper. In a large, heavy skillet, slowly heat oil, 1/8-inch deep, until very hot but not smoking. For each pancake, drop 2 tablespoons potato mixture into hot fat. With spatula, flatten against bottom of skillet to make a pancake 4 inches in diameter. Fry 2 or 3 minutes on each side or until golden brown. Drain well on paper towels. Serve hot with applesauce or sour cream. Makes 12 pancakes.

Three pancakes equal: 1/2 MEAT
1 UNSALTED STARCH (POTATO)
1 VEGETABLE

Limit to 1 Serving Potato a Day.

SCALLOPED POTATOES

1-1/2 Pounds Potatoes
2 Medium Onions
2 Tablespoons Margarine
2 Tablespoons Flour
1/4 Teaspoon Pepper
1/8 Teaspoon Paprika
1-1/2 Cups "Coffee Rich"
1 Tablespoon Parsley

Wash, pare and thinly slice potatoes (about 4 cups). Soak potatoes in water (5 times more water than potatoes) for at least 30 minutes. Drain. Cook potatoes and onions, covered in a large amount of water (5 times more water than potatoes) until slightly tender. Drain. Melt margarine in saucepan. Remove from heat. Stir in flour, pepper and paprika. Blend in "Coffee Rich". Cook over medium heat, stirring until thick and smooth.

Layer one third of the potatoes and onions in a lightly greased 2-quart casserole, sprinkle with half the parsley, top with one third of the sauce. Repeat. Add remaining potatoes and onions, top with remaining sauce. Bake at 400° uncovered for 35 minutes or until top is browned and potatoes are tender when pierced with a fork. Makes eight 1/2 cup servings.

Each serving equals: **1 UNSALTED STARCH (POTATO)**
                                1 SALTED FAT

Limit to 1 Serving Potato a Day.

SPICED SQUASH

One 12-Ounce Package Frozen Winter Squash
1 Tablespoon Margarine
Sugar Substitute to Equal 1 Tablespoon Sugar
1/4 Teaspoon Grated Orange Peel
1/8 Teaspoon Cinnamon
Dash Cloves
Dash Nutmeg

Heat squash in top of double boiler until hot. Add margarine, sugar substitute, orange peel, cinnamon, cloves and nutmeg. Stir until well blended. Makes four 1/3-cup servings.

Each serving equals: **1 VEGETABLE**

MIXED VEGETABLE SAUTE

2 Tablespoons Margarine
2 Cups Sliced Zucchini
1/2 Cup Diced Green Pepper
1/8 Teaspoon Garlic Powder
1-1/2 Cup Sliced Fresh Mushrooms
1/8 Teaspoon Pepper

Heat margarine in skillet. Saute zucchini, green pepper and garlic powder in margarine until vegetables are almost tender, stirring occasionally. Add mushrooms and pepper; saute about 10 minutes longer, stirring occasionally until vegetables are tender. Makes six 1/4-cup servings.

Each serving equals: 1 VEGETABLE

ZUCCHINI ITALIAN STYLE

1 Tablespoon Oil
1 Tablespoon Chopped Onion
1/8 Teaspoon Garlic Powder
1/2 Teaspoon Rosemary
4 Cups Sliced Zucchini
2-4 Tablespoons Water
1 Teaspoon Lemon Juice

Cook onion, garlic and rosemary in oil until onion is tender. Add zucchini and 2 to 4 tablespoons water. Cook 10 minutes just until tender. Blend in lemon juice, toss lightly. Makes six 1/2-cup servings.

Each serving equals: 1 VEGETABLE

MEXICAN RICE

3 Tablespoons Margarine
1-1/4 Cups Long Grain Rice
1/2 Cup Chopped Onion
1/4 Cup Diced Green Pepper
1/8 Teaspoon Garlic Powder
2-1/2 Cups Hot Water

One 1-Pound Can
  Low-Sodium Tomatoes
2 Teaspoons Chili Powder
1/4 Teaspoon Basil
1/4 Teaspoon Oregano
1/8 Teaspoon Pepper

Melt margarine in a large saucepan. Add rice, onion, green pepper and garlic powder. Cook, stirring, over low heat until rice browns. Add hot water, tomatoes, chili powder, basil, oregano and pepper. Bring to a boil. Cover and cook over low heat until liquid is absorbed and rice is tender, about 35 minutes. Makes seven 3/4-cup servings.

Each serving equals: 1 UNSALTED STARCH
                             1 VEGETABLE

MUSHROOM PILAF

2 Cups Fresh Sliced Mushrooms
1/2 Cup Chopped Onion
1/4 Teaspoon Garlic Powder
1 Tablespoon Parsley
1/2 Teaspoon Basil

1/8 Teaspoon Pepper
2 Tablespoons Margarine
2/3 Cup Long Grain Rice
1-1/3 Cup Water

Saute mushrooms and onions with garlic powder, parsley, basil and pepper in margarine, about 5 minutes, stirring frequently. Stir in rice and water. Cover and reduce heat. Simmer until liquid is absorbed and rice is tender, about 25 minutes. Makes four 3/4-cup servings.

Each serving equals: 1 UNSALTED STARCH
                             1 VEGETABLE
                             1/2 SALTED FAT

SALADS

APPLE GRAPE SALAD

2 Cups Diced Tart Apples, Unpeeled
2 Teaspoons Lemon Juice
3/4 Cup Diced Celery
3/4 Cup Halved, Seeded Grapes
1/4 Cup Mayonnaise
1/2 Cup "Cool Whip"

Sprinkle diced apples with lemon juice. Combine with celery, grapes and mayonnaise. Fold in "Cool Whip" and chill. Makes six 1/2-cup servings.

Each serving equals: **1 FRUIT**
                             1/2 SALTED FAT

MARINATED BEAN SALAD

One 9-Ounce Package Frozen Green Beans
One 9-Ounce Package Frozen Yellow Beans
1/4 Cup Chopped Onion
1/2 Cup Distilled Vinegar
1/2 Cup Oil
1/2 Teaspoon Pepper
1/4 Cup Chopped Green Pepper
Sugar Substitute to Equal 1/3 Cup Sugar
1/4 Teaspoon Dry Mustard

Cook beans and drain. Combine onions, vinegar, oil, pepper, green pepper, sugar substitute and dry mustard; pour over beans. Cover and allow to marinate in refrigerator overnight. Makes six 2/3-cup servings.

Each serving equals: **1 VEGETABLE**

PICKLED BEETS

1/2 Cup Vinegar
1/4 Cup Water
Sugar Substitute to Equal 1/4 Cup Sugar
3 Whole Cloves
5 Black Peppercorns
2 Tablespoons Thin Onion Slices
2 Cups Low-Sodium, Canned Beets, Drained

Combine vinegar, water, sugar substitute, cloves, peppercorns and onion slices in a saucepan. Add beets and bring to a boil. Serve hot or cold. Makes four 1/2-cup servings.

Each serving equals: 1 VEGETABLE

PINEAPPLE COLESLAW

1 Cup Finely Sliced Cabbage
1/2 Cup Drained Crushed Unsweetened Pineapple
1/2 Cup "Cool Whip"
1/4 Cup Mayonnaise

Combine cabbage and pineapple. Combine "Cool Whip" and mayonnaise. Fold into cabbage mixture. Makes four servings.

**Each serving equals: 1/2 FRUIT
                          1 SALTED FAT**

TANGY COLESLAW

6 Cups Shredded Cabbage
1 Medium Carrot, Shredded
1/2 Medium Green Pepper, Chopped
Sugar Substitute to Equal 3 Tablespoons Sugar
1/4 Cup Vinegar
2 Tablespoons Light Corn Syrup
2 Tablespoons Oil
1/4 Teaspoon Celery Seed
Dash Garlic Powder
Dash Onion Powder

Mix together cabbage, carrot and green pepper. Mix together sugar substitute, vinegar, corn syrup, oil, celery seed, garlic and onion powder. Pour over cabbage mixture and marinate overnight. Makes 8 servings.

Each serving equals: 1 VEGETABLE

CREAMY CUCUMBER SALAD

3 Cups Thinly Sliced Cucumbers
1 Cup Thinly Sliced Red Onions
1/2 Cup Mayonnaise
1 Tablespoon Parsley
1 Teaspoon Lemon Juice
1/2 Teaspoon Sugar

Add mayonnaise, parsley, lemon juice and sugar to cucumbers and onions. Toss well. Makes 6 servings.

Each serving equals: **1 VEGETABLE**
                                                 1 SALTED FAT

SWEDISH CUCUMBERS

2 Cups Sliced Cucumbers
2 Tablespoons Vinegar
1/2 Cup Sour Cream
1 Teaspoon Dill Seed
1-2 Drops "Tabasco" Sauce
1 Tablespoon Vinegar
2 Tablespoons Chopped Chives
Dash Pepper

Sprinkle cucumbers with 2 tablespoons vinegar. Let stand 30 minutes. Drain thoroughly. Combine remaining ingredients, pour over cucumbers. Chill about 30 minutes. Makes four 1/2-cup servings.

Each serving equals: **1 VEGETABLE**

MACARONI VEGETABLE SALAD

1 Cup Uncooked Elbow Macaroni
1/4 Cup Chopped Celery
2 Tablespoons Green Pepper
2 Tablespoons Shredded Carrot
2 Tablespoons Minced Onion
1/8 Teaspoon Pepper
2/3 Cup Mayonnaise
1/2 Teaspoon Sugar
1 Tablespoon Lemon Juice

Cook macaroni in unsalted boiling water according to package directions, drain. Mix macaroni, celery, green pepper, carrot, onions and pepper. Stir in mayonnaise, sugar and lemon juice; chill. Makes eight 1/3-cup servings.

Each serving equals: **1 UNSALTED STARCH**
1 SALTED FAT

TUNA MACARONI SALAD

Add one 6-1/2-ounce can Low-Sodium tuna and one chopped hard boiled egg to macaroni vegetable salad (above). Makes four 3/4-cup servings.

Each serving equals: **2 OUNCES MEAT**
1 UNSALTED STARCH
1 SALTED FAT

HOT 'N HEARTY POTATO SALAD

4 Cups Special Potatoes, Cooked
1 Cup Chopped Onion
1 Tablespoon Margarine
1-1/2 Cups Mayonnaise

1/3 Cup Vinegar
1 Tablespoon Sugar
1/4 Teaspoon Pepper
1 Teaspoon Parsley

To prepare special potatoes, peel potatoes and slice into thin slices; soak in large amount of water (5 quarts) for at least two hours or overnight, drain and cook in a large amount of water (5 quarts) until tender; drain.

In a large skillet over medium heat, cook onions in margarine 2 to 3 minutes. Stir in mayonnaise, vinegar, sugar and pepper. Add potatoes; continue cooking, stirring constantly, about 2 minutes or until heated through. DO NOT BOIL! Garnish with parsley. Makes six servings, 3/4-cup each.

**Each serving equals: 1 UNSALTED STARCH (POTATO)
2 SALTED FATS**

Limit to 1 Serving Potato a Day.

POTATO SALAD

2 Cups Special Potatoes
2 Tablespoons Minced Onion
1/4 Cup Diced Celery
1/4 Cup Diced Green Pepper
1/8 Teaspoon Regular Horseradish
1/8 Teaspoon Dry Mustard Powder
2 Teaspoons Vinegar
1/8 Teaspoon Pepper
Dash Garlic Powder
3/4 Cup Mayonnaise

To prepare special potatoes, peel potatoes and dice into small cubes. Soak in large amount of water (10 cups) for at least two hours or overnight. Drain and cook in a large amount of water (10 cups) until tender; drain and cool.

Mix potatoes, onion, celery and green pepper together lightly. Mix horseradish, mustard, vinegar, pepper, garlic powder and mayonnaise together. Pour over potato mixture, toss lightly to mix. Sprinkle with parsley or paprika. Makes 3 servings, 3/4-cup each.

Each serving equals: 1 UNSALTED STARCH (POTATO)
2 SALTED FATS

Limit to 1 Serving Potato a Day.

WALDORF SALAD

2-1/2 Cups Diced Apples, Unpeeled
1 Cup Diced Celery
1/3 Cup "Cool Whip"
2/3 Cup Mayonnaise

Combine apples and celery, fold in "Cool Whip" and mayonnaise. Makes six 1/2-cup servings.

Each serving equals: **1 FRUIT**
                              1 SALTED FAT

SALAD DRESSINGS, SAUCES, RELISHES AND SHAKERS

BLUE CHEESE DRESSING

3/4 Cup Oil
1/4 Cup Vinegar
Dash Garlic Powder
Dash Pepper
1/4 Cup Crumbled Blue Cheese

Mix oil, vinegar, garlic and pepper. Chill. Add blue cheese and toss with salad just before serving. Makes 1 cup dressing.

Limit to 2 Tablespoons a Day.

CELERY SEED DRESSING

1 Cup Oil
1/3 Cup Vinegar
1/2 Cup Confectioners' Sugar
1 Teaspoon Celery Seed
1 Teaspoon Dry Mustard
1 Teaspoon Instant Minced Onion

Place all ingredients in a jar and shake well. Refrigerate. Makes 1-1/3 cups.

Limit to 2 Tablespoons a Day.

CREAMY ITALIAN DRESSING

3/4 Cup Mayonnaise

1 Tablespoon Red Wine Vinegar

1 Tablespoon Lemon Juice

1 Tablespoon Oil

1 Tablespoon Water

1/2 Teaspoon Oregano

1 Teaspoon Sugar

1/8 Teaspoon Garlic Powder

Combine all ingredients. Chill. Makes 1 cup.

Three tablespoons equal: 1 SALTED FAT

CREAMY ROQUEFORT DRESSING

1/2 Cup Mayonnaise

1/2 Cup Sour Cream

3 Tablespoons Milk

2 Tablespoons Lemon Juice

1/4 Teaspoon Paprika

1/3 Cup Crumbled Roquefort (or Blue) Cheese

Combine all ingredients. Makes 1-1/2 cups.

Two tablespoons equal: 1 SALTED FAT

Limit to 2 Tablespoons a Day.

PARISIAN DRESSING

1 Cup Mayonnaise

1/4 Cup Oil

1/3 Cup Red Wine Vinegar

2 Tablespoons Sugar

1 Teaspoon Paprika

1/2 Teaspoon Dry Mustard

Dash Garlic

Beat oil into mayonnaise. Add remaining ingredients and stir. Makes 1-1/2 cups.

One tablespoon equals: 1 SALTED FAT

CACCIATORE SAUCE

1/2 Cup Thinly Sliced Onions
1/2 Cup Diced Fresh Mushrooms
1 Tablespoon Margarine
1/8 Teaspoon Garlic Powder
1 Cup Low-Sodium Canned Tomatoes, Chopped
2 Tablespoons Tomato Paste (Canned Without Salt)
1/8 Teaspoon Pepper
1/2 Teaspoon Oregano
1/4 Teaspoon Basil
1 Bay Leaf
1/4 Cup Red Wine
2 Teaspoons Cornstarch
1/2 Cup Water

Melt margarine in a large skillet. Saute onions and mushrooms with garlic powder in margarine until onions are transparent. Add the remaining ingredients, cover and simmer for 1 hour. Serve as a sauce over fish, veal or chicken (which has been baked or broiled with an herb flavored margarine) with noodles or rice on the side. Makes 2 cups.

One-third cup equals: 1 VEGETABLE

CUCUMBER SAUCE

1/2 Small Unpeeled Cucumber
1 Cup Sour Cream
1 Teaspoon Dill Weed
1 Teaspoon Instant Minced Onion
1/4 Teaspoon Pepper

Shred cucumber, add remaining ingredients and mix. Refrigerate. Serve with tuna, salmon or other fish. Makes 1 cup.

One-quarter cup equals: 1/2 VEGETABLE

HERBED MARGARINE

1/4 Cup Margarine
1 Teaspoon Marjoram
1/8 Teaspoon Basil
1/8 Teaspoon Parsley
1 Teaspoon Dill Weed
1/2 Teaspoon Onion Powder
1/8 Teaspoon Garlic Powder
1/4 Teaspoon Paprika

Cream margarine until soft. In another bowl crush all the herbs against the side of the bowl with a spoon. Sprinkle the crushed herbs into the margarine and mix. Spread on bread, serve over vegetables or melt and pour over popcorn. Makes 1/4 cup.

One tablespoon equals: 1 SALTED FAT

NOTE: Herbs can be adjusted to individual taste.

HOLLANDAISE SAUCE

3 Egg Yolks
2 Tablespoons Lemon Juice
Dash "Tabasco" Sauce
1/2 Cup Hot, Bubbling Margarine

Put egg yolks, lemon juice and "Tabasco" in blender or food processor. Cover. Blend egg yolk mixture about 5 seconds, then add hot margarine in a steady stream, while continuing to blend. Blend until thick, about 30 seconds. Serve immediately over asparagus, broccoli, poached eggs, croquettes or fish. Makes 3/4 cup.

1-1/2 tablespoons equal: 1 SALTED FAT

Limit to 1 Serving a Day.

MOCK HOLLANDAISE SAUCE

2 Tablespoons Hot Water
1/2 Cup Mayonnaise
1 Tablespoon Lemon Juice
Yellow Food Coloring

Blend hot water into mayonnaise in top of double boiler until blended and heated through. (Use wire whisk to blend.) Add lemon juice and a drop of yellow food coloring. Makes 2/3 cup.

Three tablespoons equal: 1 SALTED FAT

SOUR CREAM SAUCE

2 Tablespoons Margarine
2 Tablespoons Chopped Onions
1/2 Cup Sour Cream
Dash Pepper

Saute onion in margarine until tender. Stir in sour cream and heat through. Do not boil. Serve over or mix with hot cooked vegetables. Sprinkle with parsley, if desired. Makes 1/2 cup.

Two tablespoons equal: 1 SALTED FAT

Limit to 1 Serving a Day.

VINAIGRETTE SAUCE

1/4 Cup Lemon Juice
1/2 Teaspoon Pepper
1/8 Teaspoon Garlic Powder
1/4 Teaspoon Dry Mustard

2 Tablespoons Vinegar
5 Tablespoons Oil
1 Tablespoon Sour Cream

Combine all ingredients and shake well. Pour over hot cooked vegetables or use as a marinade for chilled vegetables. Makes 3/4 cup.

Each serving is free.

HOT MUSTARD

2/3 Cup Dry Mustard
1/4 Cup Sugar
1/4 Cup Oil
1/2 Cup Wine Vinegar
1/2 Cup Water

Combine all ingredients; blend well. Refrigerate. Makes 1-1/2 cups.

Each serving is FREE

ZIPPY MAYONNAISE

Mix equal parts of mayonnaise and hot mustard.

Two tablespoons of
Zippy Mayonnaise equal: 1 SALTED FAT

SOUTH OF THE BORDER RELISH

1 Cup Finely Diced Tomatoes
1/2 Cup Minced Onion
1/2 Cup Finely Chopped Hot Peppers
  (Or Sweet Red Peppers, If Desired)
2 Teaspoons Vinegar
1/8 Teaspoon Garlic Powder
1/8 Teaspoon Grated Lemon Peel
1 Teaspoon Lemon Juice
"Tabasco" Sauce to Taste

Combine ingredients. Cover and refrigerate 8 hours. Makes 2 cups.

One tablespoon is FREE

Limit to 1 Tablespoons a Day.

DILL PICKLES

4 Pounds Cucumbers (4-Inches Long)
3 Cups Distilled Vinegar
3 Cups Water
3/4 to 1 Cup Dill Seed
18-21 Whole Black Peppercorns

Wash and slice cucumbers. Heat vinegar and water to boiling. Pack cucumbers into pint jars. Add 2 tablespoons dill seed and 3 peppercorns to each jar. Fill to within 1/2-inch of the top with boiling vinegar liquid. Seal and process in boiling water bath 20 minutes. Makes 6 pints.

Two tablespoons are FREE

HERB SHAKER FOR MEATS

1/4 Cup Parsley

1 Tablespoon Basil

1 Tablespoon Oregano

1 Tablespoon Paprika

1 Teaspoon Celery Flakes

Sprinkle herbs into blender. Set on low. Blend until well powdered. Store in airtight container.

SALAD HERBS

1/4 Cup Parsley

1/4 Cup Tarragon

1 Tablespoon Oregano

1 Teaspoon Dried Dill Weed

1 Tablespoon Celery Flakes

Sprinkle into blender set on low. Blend until well powdered. Store in airtight container.

HERB BLEND

1 Teaspoon Basil

1 Teaspoon Marjoram

1 Teaspoon Thyme

1 Teaspoon Oregano

1 Teaspoon Parsley

1 Teaspoon Nutmeg

1 Teaspoon Pepper

1/2 Teaspoon Savory

1/2 Teaspoon Ground Cloves

1/2 Teaspoon Cayenne

Combine and store in airtight container.

EACH SERVING IS FREE

NUTRITIVE VALUES OF RECIPES

RECIPE	Servings	Calories	Protein gm	Fat gm	Carbohy-drate, gm	Sodium mg	Potassium mg
Almond Flavored Shortbread	14	3080	31.0	187	320	2246	328
	1	220	2.2	13	23	161	23
Apple Cheese-Filled Rolls	18	2829	48.5	168	309	1790	754
	1	157	2.7	9	17	99	42
Apple Grape Salad	6	740	2.6	53	68	455	817
	1	123	0.4	9	11	76	136
Apple Muffins	16	2042	36.9	72	315	770	1178
	1	128	2.3	5	20	48	74
Baked Crab Imperial	6	1754	117.6	94	99	2892	2149
	1	292	19.6	16	17	482	358
Baking Powder Biscuits	12	1715	35.1	76	220	968	523
	1	143	2.9	6	18	81	44
Banana Split Dessert	9	1989	15.9	115	230	1507	1134
	1	221	1.8	13	26	167	126
Beef Ragout	5	1177	94.6	79	19	620	1817
	1	235	18.9	16	4	124	363
Beef Steak with Onions	6	1461	100.8	92	57	778	2074
	1	244	16.8	15	10	130	346
Beef Stroganoff	6	2283	150.3	168	34	604	2970
	1	381	25.0	28	6	101	495
Beef Coating Recipe	6	404	13.0	5	76	746	238
	1	67	2.2	1	13	124	40
Biscuit Mix	3-3/4 cups	2108	43.2	71	318	2109	390
Blueberry Cake Muffins	18	2987	48.0	112	455	1748	737
	1	166	2.7	6	25	97	41
Blueberry Kuchen	16	2216	33.0	81	314	1549	597
	1	139	2.1	5	20	97	37
Blueberry Pancakes	10	1235	30.9	51	165	1188	690
	1	124	3.1	5	17	119	69
Blue Cheese Dressing	16	1576	7.2	174	4	481	47
	1	99	0.5	11	-	30	3

RECIPE	Servings	Calories	Protein gm	Fat gm	Carbohy-drate, gm	Sodium mg	Potassium mg
Breaded Veal Cutlets	6	2272	113.4	168	76	1423	1732
	1	379	18.9	28	13	237	288
Broiled Fish	1 oz.	66	7.1	4	-	75	159
Brownie Mix	16 cups	11427	89.7	432	2061	3517	3757
Brownies	12	2273	25.8	134	261	1318	682
	1	189	2.2	11	22	110	57
Cacciatore Sauce	6	284	5.7	13	34	174	1124
	1	47	1.0	2	6	29	187
Carrots Vichy	4	305	3.1	24	23	387	706
	1	76	0.8	6	6	97	177
Celery Seed Dressing	10	2169	-	218	64	6	78
	1	217	-	22	6	1	8
Chicken Breasts and Mushrooms in Wine	8	888	122.4	36	11	542	2164
	1	111	15.3	5	1	68	271
Chicken Cacciatore	5	1172	90.1	72	34	966	2111
	1	234	18.0	14	7	193	422
Chicken Coating Recipe	6	403	13.0	5	75	746	240
	1	67	2.2	1	13	124	40
Chicken Croquettes	7	2843	122.3	192	152	1910	1908
	1	406	17.5	27	22	273	273
Chicken Noodle Casserole	6	2656	100.5	176	164	1751	1107
	1	443	16.8	24	27	292	185
Chicken N' Orange Salad	3	849	47.0	64	25	618	1012
	1	283	15.7	21	8	206	337
Chicken Paprikash	6	1269	95.4	79	38	695	1912
	1	212	15.9	13	6	116	319
Chicken with Wine and Grapes	5	1354	86.6	83	56	1082	1424
	1	271	17.3	17	11	216	285
Chopped Chicken Livers	7	1545	111.7	102	32	1273	1412
	1	221	16.0	15	5	182	202
Christmas Slices	18	3373	38.5	193	374	2309	413
	1	184	2.1	11	20	126	23

RECIPE	Servings	Calories	Protein gm	Fat gm	Carbohy-drate, gm	Sodium mg	Potassium mg
Corn Muffins	18	1828	40.3	72	251	1237	712
	1	102	2.2	4	14	69	40
Coquilles St. Jacques	3	908	49.5	59	43	1357	1575
	1	303	16.5	20	14	452	525
Crab Rice Casserole	6	2046	111.3	117	126	2361	1777
	1	341	18.6	20	21	394	296
Cranberry Nut Pudding	8	2194	21.1	104	268	955	1036
	1	274	2.6	13	34	119	130
Creamy Cucumber Salad	6	941	7.5	88	36	705	986
	1	157	1.3	15	6	118	164
Creamy Italian Dressing	5	1329	2.0	146	10	985	107
	1	266	0.4	29	2	185	20
Creamy Roquefort Dressing	12	1220	16.1	126	11	1368	272
	1	102	1.3	11	1	114	23
Cucumber Sauce	4	471	7.6	43	11	105	333
	1	118	1.9	11	3	26	83
Curried Corn	4	421	8.5	27	52	564	545
	1	105	2.1	7	13	141	136
Dill Pickles	96	596	34.6	2	140	1194	3912
	1	6	0.4	-	1	12	41
Dilled Green Beans	3	312	5.7	23	21	293	562
	1	104	1.9	8	7	98	187
Easy Layer Cake	16	2288	29.9	78	366	1661	626
	1	143	1.9	5	23	104	39
Egg Salad	1	291	6.9	28	3	230	85
Eggplant and Ground Beef Casserole	4	1737	79.1	115	100	822	1955
	1	434	19.8	29	25	206	489
Fettuccini Alfredo	4	1456	46.3	84	129	896	450
	1	364	11.6	21	32	224	112
Fish Au Gratin	5	970	77.7	68	12	941	1738
	1	194	15.5	14	2	188	348

Flavored Coffees (see Vienna, Orange and Mocha Flavored Coffee)

RECIPE	Servings	Calories	Protein gm	Fat gm	Carbohy-drate, gm	Sodium mg	Potassium mg
French Toast	6	739	33.8	23	94	1066	567
	1	123	5.6	4	16	178	95
Fried Cabbage and Noodles	5	390	7.3	25	36	313	221
	1	78	1.5	5	7	63	44
Fried Potatoes	6	1007	14.7	62	104	782	898
	1	168	2.5	10	17	130	150
Frozen Chocolate Chip Cheesecake	10	3745	61.5	283	269	2672	1900
	1	373	6.2	28	27	267	190
German Coffee Cake	12	1810	28.4	69	269	1429	676
	1	151	2.4	6	22	119	56
Glorified Rice	8	1226	6.3	56	159	58	304
	1	153	0.8	7	20	7	38
Gourmet Green Beans	3	234	4.4	17	15	214	420
	1	78	1.5	6	5	71	140
Gourmet Hamburgers	5	1705	84.5	135	15	768	1609
	1	341	16.9	27	3	154	322
Graham Cracker Pie Crust	Whole Recipe	948	9.2	56	108	1321	454
Greenbeans and Mushrooms	4	355	6.3	29	18	364	702
	1	89	1.6	7	5	91	176
Harvard Beets	4	399	2.8	23	36	416	506
	1	100	0.7	6	9	104	127
Hawaiian Chicken Salad	4	1256	69.6	95	31	867	1498
	1	314	17.4	24	8	217	375
Hawaiian Quick Bread	20	2172	43.1	76	329	1929	654
	1	109	2.2	4	16	96	33
Hawaiian Shrimp Salad	5	1826	87.4	137	69	1786	2168
	1	365	17.5	27	14	357	434
Herb Blend	8-1/2 tsp.	33	0.9	1	4	3	190
	1/4 tsp.	1	-	-	-	-	6
Herb Shaker for Meats	7 tsp.	61	2.8	-	12	17	435
	1/2 tsp.	2	0.1	-	-	-	10
Herbed Margarine	4	419	0.9	46	2	564	86
	1	105	0.2	12	1	141	22
Holiday Cranberry Bread	20	2616	46.2	67	452	1479	1083
	1	131	2.3	3	23	74	54

RECIPE	Servings	Calories	Protein gm	Fat gm	Carbohy- drate, gm	Sodium mg	Potassium mg
Holiday Eggnog	6	808	14.2	45	82	372	258
	1	135	2.4	8	14	62	43
Hollandaise Sauce	8	999	8.9	108	3	1146	119
	1	125	1.1	14	-	143	15
Hot Cabbage Slaw	6	396	5.5	25	41	355	1019
	1	66	0.9	4	7	59	170
Hot Cocoa Mix	38	705	19.5	40	83	329	1565
	1	19	0.5	1	2	9	41
Hot Deviled Carrots	4	300	3.0	24	22	382	708
	1	75	0.8	5	6	96	177
Hot Muffins	16	1876	36.6	72	271	768	614
	1	117	2.3	5	17	48	38
Hot Mustard	1-1/2 cups	683	-	55	55	7	504
	2 tsp.	19	-	2	2	-	14
Hot Roast Beef Sandwich	8	1827	143.3	120	29	988	3091
	1	228	17.9	15	4	124	386
Hot Spiced Wine	3	317	0.2	-	40	6	466
	1	106	-	-	13	2	155
Hot N' Hearty Potato Salad	6	3001	11.9	276	127	2142	911
	1	500	2.0	46	21	357	152
Hungarian Pancakes	10 pancakes	1174	17.9	52	152	319	314
	1 pancake	117	1.8	5	15	32	31
Hungarian Pork Chops	3	877	56.4	68	7	193	746
	1	292	18.8	23	2	64	249
Impossible Pumpkin Pie	8	1701	24.2	68	249	670	1276
	1	213	3.0	9	31	84	160
Italian Pie	6	2202	125.7	126	138	1549	2733
	1	367	21.0	21	23	258	456
Italian Sausage	9	1091	69.5	88	2	172	827
	1	121	7.7	10	-	19	92
Jam Bars	14	2343	30.9	102	365	1398	744
	1	167	2.2	7	23	100	53
Jelly-Filled Muffins	16	1876	36.6	72	271	768	614
	1	117	2.3	5	17	48	38

RECIPE	Servings	Calories	Protein gm	Fat gm	Carbohy-drate, gm	Sodium mg	Potassium mg
Jelly-Roll Cake	16	1427	32.7	23	273	565	531
	1	89	2.0	1	17	35	33
Lamb Curry	5	1963	82.0	162	43	945	2061
	1	393	16.4	32	9	189	412
Lasagna	Whole Recipe	3672	240.0	186	260	2583	5081
	Cut into 12, 1 serving	306	20.0	16	22	215	423
	Cut into 9, 1 serving	408	26.7	21	29	287	565
Lemon Broiled Chicken	5 oz.	496	42.3	34	4	117	578
	1 oz.	99	8.5	7	1	23	116
Lemon Carrots	6	352	4.5	24	34	433	1057
	1	59	0.8	4	6	72	176
Lemon Drops	18	2786	42.9	108	415	1849	511
	1	155	2.4	6	23	103	28
Lemon Tea Bread	20	3214	54.2	147	424	1733	815
	1	161	2.7	7	21	87	41
Light and Fruity Pie Strawberry	8	1819	18.2	113	177	1442	1114
	1	227	2.3	14	22	180	139
Blueberry	8	1854	18.2	113	186	1442	987
	1	232	2.3	14	23	180	123
Raspberry	8	1834	18.7	113	181	1442	1077
	1	229	2.3	14	23	180	135
Pineapple	8	1953	18.0	112	214	1444	1115
	1	244	2.3	14	27	181	139
Lime Snow	8	687	19.6	-	159	96	223
	1	86	2.5	-	20	12	28
London Broil	6	716	98.1	33	-	344	1589
	1	119	16.4	6	-	57	265
Macaroni and Cheese	6	2592	106.2	139	226	2399	1385
	1	432	17.7	23	38	400	231
Macaroni Vegetable Salad	8	1495	16.9	117	94	928	463
	1	187	2.1	15	12	116	58
Marble Loaf Cake	24	3494	49.1	140	517	2455	1078
	1	146	2.0	6	22	102	45
Marinated Bean Salad	6	1125	9.0	109	38	14	932
	1	188	1.5	18	6	2	155

RECIPE	Servings	Calories	Protein gm	Fat gm	Carbohy- drate, gm	Sodium mg	Potassium mg
Meat Coatings (see Beef, Veal, Chicken or Pork Chop Meat Coatings							
Meat Loaf	8	2151	142.0	161	23	730	2398
	1	269	17.8	20	3	91	300
Meat Salads Salmon	1	286	12.0	26	2	205	225
Tuna	1	278	16.3	22	2	192	178
Chicken	1	300	18.3	24	2	205	253
Turkey	1	314	18.3	25	2	243	228
Meltaways	18	3662	36.4	272	352	2248	663
	1	203	2.0	15	20	125	37
Mexican Rice	7	1291	22.6	37	208	461	1496
	1	184	3.2	5	30	66	214
Mixed Vegetable Saute	6	304	6.9	24	17	310	1078
	1	51	1.2	4	3	52	180
Mocha Flavored Coffee	20	592	4.2	36	63	290	1590
	1	30	0.2	2	3	15	80
Mock Hollandaise Sauce	2/3 cup	793	1.3	88	3	657	59
	3 Tbsp.	223	0.4	25	1	185	17
Mushroom Pilaf	4	731	13.9	24	113	320	889
	1	183	3.5	6	28	80	222
Old-Time Country Sausage	9	1093	69.4	88	1	172	798
	1	121	7.7	10	-	19	89
Onion Parsley Butterfingers	16	2085	34.7	140	179	2374	577
	1	130	2.2	9	11	148	36
Orange Flavored Coffee	20	568	2.4	34	59	218	1540
	1	28	0.1	2	3	11	77
Osso Bucco	4	1127	71.7	77	24	778	1514
	1	282	17.9	19	6	195	378
Oven Dinner	1	450	19.0	30	28	225	565

RECIPE		Servings	Calories	Protein gm	Fat gm	Carbohy-drate, gm	Sodium mg	Potassium mg
Oven Fried Potatoes		1	208	2.6	14	20	3	200
Pancakes		10 pancakes	1144	29.7	50	142	1186	556
		1 pancake	114	3.0	5	14	119	56
Parisian Dressing		24	2152	2.7	231	30	1315	212
		1	90	0.1	10	1	55	9
Pickled Beets		4	149	3.4	-	38	159	633
		1	37	0.9	-	10	40	158
Pie Shell	2-Crust	Whole Recipe	2324	28.8	153	209	6	260
	1-Crust	Whole Recipe	1206	14.4	81	104	3	130
Pineapple Coleslaw		4	577	2.1	52	27	355	359
		1	144	0.5	13	7	89	90
Pineapple Cookies		12	1931	29.0	99	285	1208	406
		1	161	2.4	8	24	101	34
Piquant Liver and Onions		6	1220	96.1	64	62	1191	1521
		1	203	16.0	10	10	199	254
Pizza		16 slices	3459	158.3	182	296	1111	3664
		3 slices	636	29.7	33	56	208	687
		2 slices	432	19.8	22	37	139	458
Popover Pancake		2	989	24.9	63	81	745	385
		1	495	12.5	32	41	373	193
Pot Roast of Beef		8	1827	143.3	120	29	988	3091
		1	228	17.9	15	4	124	386
Pork Chops Coating Recipe		6	407	13.1	5	76	746	259
		1	68	2.2	1	13	124	43
Potato Pancakes		4	766	29.9	13	135	138	1020
		1	192	7.5	3	33	36	340
Potato Salad		3	1412	7.0	132	55	1037	498
		1	471	2.3	44	18	346	166
Pumpkin Bread		20	2533	49.0	66	435	1936	1202
		1	127	2.5	3	22	97	60
Quick Biscuits		6	615	4.3	22	89	603	221
		1	103	2.4	4	15	10	37
Quick Chocolate Ice Cream		6	632	1.7	33	79	71	244
		1	105	0.3	6	13	12	41

RECIPE	Servings	Calories	Protein gm	Fat gm	Carbohy-drate, gm	Sodium mg	Potassium mg
Rice-Stuffed Chicken	6	1370	12.0	93	123	1145	461
	1	228	2.0	16	21	191	77
Rich Almond Cookies	17	3198	37.1	197	320	2264	362
	1	190	2.2	12	19	134	22
Roast Pork with Apples and Raisins	12	3884	196.6	283	128	705	4196
	1	324	16.4	24	11	59	350
Salad Herbs	18 Tbsp.	93	5.9	-	18	32	861
	1/2 tsp.	1	0.1	-	-	-	8
Salmon Patties	6	1020	104.8	55	19	336	1704
	1	170	17.5	9	3	56	284
Sauerbraten	10	2082	163.8	144	27	1130	2757
	1	208	16.4	14	3	113	276

Sausage (see Italian, Spanish and Old-Time Country Sausage.)

RECIPE	Servings	Calories	Protein gm	Fat gm	Carbohy-drate, gm	Sodium mg	Potassium mg
Savory Brussels Sprouts	6	513	10.5	47	20	604	940
	1	86	1.8	8	3	101	157
Scrambled Potatoes and Eggs	3	1051	44.7	84	34	701	651
	1	350	14.9	28	11	234	217
Scalloped Potatoes	8	1348	19.2	58	191	514	1047
	1	169	2.4	7	24	64	131
Scottish Shortbread	16	3280	37.4	188	362	2249	383
	1	205	2.3	12	23	141	24
Seafood Quiche with Crab	6	2785	99.3	191	161	3028	1324
	1	464	16.6	32	27	504	221
with Shrimp	6	2802	105.8	190	161	2770	1479
	1	467	17.6	32	27	462	247
with Tuna	6	2826	112.5	190	160	2653	1509
	1	471	18.8	32	27	442	252
Sherried Beef Stroganoff	6	1969	107.5	123	63	852	2411
	1	328	17.9	21	11	142	402
Shish Kabob	5	1302	89.2	86	43	473	2358
	1	260	17.8	17	9	95	472
Short-Cut Brownies	16	1592	24.2	66	259	562	600
	1	100	1.5	4	16	35	38

RECIPE	Servings	Calories	Protein gm	Fat gm	Carbohy-drate, gm	Sodium mg	Potassium mg
Shrimp and Fish Creole	5	1397	98.8	17	214	641	3177
	1	279	19.8	3	43	128	635
Shrimp Broiled with Garlic Butter	5	1244	83.5	96	12	1758	1099
	1	249	16.7	19	2	352	220
Snickerdoodles	30	4476	54.2	200	616	4305	952
	1	149	1.8	7	21	144	32
Sour Cream Sauce	4	439	4.0	45	6	330	107
	1	110	1.0	11	2	83	27
South of the Border Relish	32	101	4.9	1	22	24	751
	1	3	0.2	-	1	1	23
Spaghetti Sauce	8	2235	133.5	158	70	552	4615
	1	279	16.7	20	9	69	577
Spanish Sausage	9	1116	70.0	88	5	202	827
	1	124	7.8	10	1	22	92
Spiced French Toast	6	743	33.8	23	95	1066	576
	1	124	5.6	4	16	178	96
Spiced Squash	4	252	4.2	13	32	143	711
	1	63	1.1	3	8	36	178
Spiced Tea	24	70	2.8	-	16	1	1109
	1	3	0.1	-	1	-	46
Strawberry Cream Cheese Pie	10	2525	29.4	175	218	1914	1147
	1	253	2.9	18	22	191	115
Streusel-Topped Muffins	14	2159	34.2	81	326	1420	703
	1	154	2.4	6	23	101	50
Stuffed Cabbage Rolls	6	1789	106.3	109	93	506	3123
	1	298	17.7	18	16	84	521
Stuffed Flank Steak	9	1850	160.3	100	60	1698	3360
	1	206	17.8	11	7	189	373
Stuffed Pepper Cups	5	1863	101.7	99	136	541	3277
	1	373	20.3	20	27	108	655
Swedish Cucumbers	4	280	6.2	22	16	68	602
	1	70	1.6	6	4	17	151
Sweet Chocolate Cream Pie	10	2459	23.6	163	236	1643	971
	1	246	2.4	16	24	164	97

RECIPE	Servings	Calories	Protein gm	Fat gm	Carbohy- drate, gm	Sodium mg	Potassium mg
Tangy Coleslaw	8	561	7.2	29	68	182	1403
	1	70	0.9	4	9	23	176
Tea Cakes	16	2913	31.7	187	200	2247	336
	1	182	2.0	12	13	140	21
Texas Cake	30	3436	49.2	87	623	1942	806
	1	115	1.6	3	21	65	27
Thumbprint Cookies	8	1645	15.9	98	154	1138	231
	1	206	2.0	12	19	142	29
Tropical Cheesecake	8	2330	23.8	146	242	1174	984
	1	291	3.0	18	30	147	123
Tuna Croquettes	7	2729	141.3	170	152	1906	2172
	1	390	20.2	24	22	272	310
Tuna Macaroni Salad	4	1807	74.7	126	94	1063	1025
	1	452	18.7	32	24	266	256
Tuna Noodle Casserole	6	2614	110.0	166	164	1749	1241
	1	436	18.3	28	27	292	207
Tuna Patties	8	736	118.4	17	19	276	1218
	1	92	14.8	2	2	35	152
Tuna Rice Casserole	6	1963	103.9	113	124	1188	1366
	1	327	17.3	19	21	198	228
Turkey Broccoli Au Gratin	6	1461	110.1	89	52	1344	1993
	1	244	18.4	15	9	224	332
Turkey Croquettes	7	2793	126.5	184	152	2120	2174
	1	399	18.1	26	22	303	310
Turkey Glory Sandwich	6	2514	111.1	169	132	2543	1236
	1	419	18.5	28	22	424	206
Turkey Noodle Casserole	6	2611	104.6	169	164	1789	1303
	1	435	17.4	28	27	298	217
Veal Coating	6	404	13.0	5	76	746	238
	1	67	2.2	1	13	124	40
Veal Goulash	6	1601	97.4	113	43	944	2100
	1	267	16.2	19	7	157	350
Veal Picatta	3	578	58.2	38	8	362	810
	1	193	19.4	13	3	121	270

RECIPE	Servings	Calories	Protein gm	Fat gm	Carbohy- drate, gm	Sodium mg	Potassium mg
Veal with Sour Cream	6	2119	103.6	156	37	854	2162
	1	353	17.3	26	6	142	360
Vegetable Fish Bake	6	1057	93.7	52	50	1120	2242
	1	176	15.6	9	8	187	374
Vienna Flavored Coffee	20	376	1.6	22	38	141	1024
	1	19	0.1	1	2	7	51
Vinaigrette Sauce	6	652	0.9	71	8	8	118
	1	121	0.1	12	1	1	20
Waldorf Salad	6	1308	3.6	124	53	1034	767
	1	218	0.6	21	9	172	128
Western Gingerbread	24	3265	44.8	122	501	2958	1207
	1	136	1.9	5	21	123	50
Zippy Mayonnaise	2 Tbsp.	127	0.2	13	3	82	26
Zucchini Bread	20	3124	46.0	158	400	887	1169
	1	156	2.3	8	20	44	58
Zucchini Italian Style	6	224	5.8	15	18	7	962
	1	37	1.0	3	3	1	160

INDEX

INDEX

INDEX

INDEX

INDEX